THE

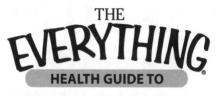

EVERYTHING

HEALTH GUIDE TO

LIVING WITH BREAST CANCER

Dear Reader,

You just heard the dreaded news. You have breast cancer. Now what? Where do you begin? Your mind races through emotions and thoughts so quickly that you can't get a handle on them. You feel overwhelmed and wonder whether you are going to make the right choices. You are bombarded with medical information and are trying to make sense of it. At the same time, you are too upset to think about your medical treatment options in a rational way.

You feel a sense of urgency, you can't understand why you have breast cancer and you wonder what went wrong. You ask, "Why is my body failing me?" These are some of the questions and concerns that come with the diagnosis of breast cancer. It challenges your concept of self, what your breasts mean to you, and the importance you place on your body image.

I have been living with the diagnosis of breast cancer for sixteen years. At the time of my diagnosis, I was working on an oncology unit at a major hospital. Even so, I found myself, a nurse, overwhelmed with the diagnosis and the many treatment options that came with it. This is what fueled my desire to start a local walk called "The Rays of Hope Walk Toward the Cure of Breast Cancer," which has given many local women and men the resources, education, and support they need. My hope is that this guide will give you the information that you need to make an informed decision about your breast cancer treatment, because an informed decision is always a go͏

Lucy Giuggio Carvalho

WELCOME TO THE

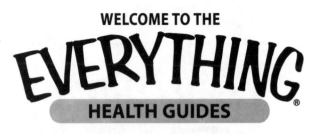

EVERYTHING

HEALTH GUIDES

Everything® Health Guides are a part of the bestselling *Everything®* series and cover important health topics like anxiety, postpartum care, and thyroid disease. Packed with the most recent, up-to-date data, *Everything®* Health Guides help you get the right diagnosis, choose the best doctor, and find the treatment options that work for you. With this one comprehensive resource, you and your family members have all the information you need right at your fingertips.

 Alerts

Urgent warnings

 Facts

Important snippets of information

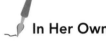 **Essentials**

Quick handy tips

 Questions

Answers to common questions

In Her Own Words

Quotes from real-life survivors/family members

When you're done reading, you can finally say you know **EVERYTHING®**!

PUBLISHER Karen Cooper

DIRECTOR OF ACQUISITIONS AND INNOVATION Paula Munier

MANAGING EDITOR, EVERYTHING® SERIES Lisa Laing

COPY CHIEF Casey Ebert

ACQUISITIONS EDITOR Katrina Schroeder

DEVELOPMENT EDITOR Brett Palana-Shanahan

EDITORIAL ASSISTANT Hillary Thompson

EVERYTHING® SERIES COVER DESIGNER Erin Alexander

LAYOUT DESIGNERS Colleen Cunningham, Elisabeth Lariviere, Ashley Vierra, Denise Wallace

Visit the entire Everything® series at *www.everything.com*

THE EVERYTHING®
HEALTH GUIDE TO
LIVING WITH
BREAST
CANCER

An accessible and comprehensive
resource for women

Lucia Giuggio Carvalho, RN, MSN
and James A. Stewart, MD

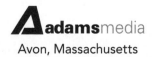

Avon, Massachusetts

*To all the Rays of Hope Walkers in Western
Massachusetts and to all those who have been touched
by breast cancer. We will never lose hope for a cure.*

An Everything® Series Book.
Everything® and everything.com® are registered trademarks of F+W Media, Inc.

Published by Adams Media, a division of F+W Media, Inc.
57 Littlefield Street, Avon, MA 02322 U.S.A.
www.adamsmedia.com

ISBN 10: 1-59869-921-0
ISBN 13: 978-1-59869-921-0

Printed in the United States of America.

J I H G F E D C B A

Library of Congress Cataloging-in-Publication Data
is available from the publisher.

This publication is designed to provide accurate and authoritative information with
regard to the subject matter covered. It is sold with the understanding that the publisher is not engaged in rendering legal, accounting, or other professional advice.
If legal advice or other expert assistance is required, the services of a competent
professional person should be sought.
—From a *Declaration of Principles* jointly adopted by a Committee of the
American Bar Association and a Committee of Publishers and Associations

Many of the designations used by manufacturers and sellers to distinguish their
products are claimed as trademarks. Where those designations appear in this book
and Adams Media was aware of a trademark claim, the designations have been
printed with initial capital letters.

*This book is available at quantity discounts for bulk purchases.
For information, please call 1-800-289-0963.*

All the examples and dialogues used in this book are fictional, and
have been created by the author to illustrate disciplinary situations.

Acknowledgments

Thanks from the bottom of my heart:

To my loving and supportive husband, Jim Carvalho; my step-children, Alicia and Kyle; my sister, Connie Torcia and her family; the Giuggio family; and the Mazzaferro family. To Enza Valenti, Marie Jablonski, Joan Sirard, Holly Joy Denis, Susanne McGlynn, Linda Donoghue, Mary Lou Cross, Irina Loban, Karen Johnson, Dr. Paul Hetzel, Dr. William Reed, Dr. Grace Makari-Judson, Sandra Hubbard, Marlene Quinlan, Susan Dugan, Dr. Brian Acker, Kathy Tobin, Deb Levy, my church group friends (Elaine Bloniasz, Phyllis LeFleur, Carolee Arsenault, Bill Whitney), the "ladies guild" (Marian Broder, Gale Kirkwood, Carol Baribeau), Baystate Medical Center, the Comprehensive Breast Center, the Rays of Hope Steering Committee, the Comprehensive Breast Center Community Advisory Board, Gaetana M. Aliotta, and the Cancer House of Hope, Cancer Connection, and my golden retriever, Sophie.

And all those—too many to mention—who will always remain in my heart, especially all those who have walked before me and those who will walk behind me on their breast cancer journey until there is a cure.

Contents

Introduction

The *Everything® Health Guide to Living with Breast Cancer* comes from the firsthand experience of a sixteen-year survivor. It provides a basic overview of breast cancer, its biology, psychology, and treatment options, along with the practical and spiritual advice needed to get through treatment. It is a holistic approach to facing breast cancer with your mind, body, and spirit. It covers the physical changes that occur with treatment, such as hair loss, early menopause, fatigue, sexuality, weight gain/loss, as well as support systems, medical insurance coverage, financial considerations, complementary and alternative medicine choices, and more.

This guide provides newly diagnosed individuals and their families with an overview of the physical, psychological, and emotional aspects of dealing with a breast cancer diagnosis and the journey associated with it. It also addresses the spiritual and philosophical elements of going through this journey. The guide will also help you to explore ways to take an inventory of your past life and will empower you to live in the moment and decide how you want to live the rest of your life. It teaches you about participating in and enjoying each day, no matter where you are in your breast cancer journey. This guide also incorporates humor and fun into the experience.

Researchers are making great strides in the diagnosis and treatment of breast cancer, from studying the molecular biology of cancer, targeting specific breast cancer cells in treatment of certain cancers, understanding how cells divide and looking at the proteins/genes that contribute to cell growth and cell death. Most recently, researchers are looking at alternatives or adjuncts to traditional mammography and magnetic resonance imaging (MRI) that could possibly be more effective. Current cancer treatment focus is on controlling growth of existing tumors and preventing their spread. Combination treatment using chemotherapy, radiation, surgery, and antibody and hormonal therapies is being explored. Scientists are also trying to develop vaccines that would prevent breast cancer, though this approach needs much more work.

This is not an all-knowing, finite, authoritative book about how to live with breast cancer. There is no answer as to why one person is a breast cancer survivor and another is not. The breast cancer journey is not about doing everything right for the right outcome. Some see their diagnosis of breast cancer as a one-time event and some see it as a lifelong experience. However you view your breast cancer experience, it is yours to view, to hold, to feel deep within your soul. It is about living life in whatever stage of your breast cancer treatment you are in and to find within yourself the strength, courage, and spirit to live with it.

CHAPTER 1

An Overview
of Breast Cancer

What is breast cancer? Cells normally develop, grow, multiply, and die in all tissues, including the breast. Breast cancer occurs when cells divide out of control and the mechanism that usually regulates cell division is not working. In the most common types of breast cancer, it is thought that cancer cells begin either in the ducts or the lobular tissue of the breast. Cancer cells multiply and form a lump, or mass, called a tumor. The cells can also invade and destroy healthy tissue. Cells from a cancerous tumor in the breast can break away and spread to other organs in the body, a process known as metastasis.

Risk Factors for Breast Cancer

The major risk factor for breast cancer is being a woman. Only 1 percent of breast cancer occurs in men. Some other known risk factors for breast cancer include: family history of the disease, especially in one's mother or sister (it is important to remember that an inherited risk of developing breast cancer can come from the mother's side and also the father's side, so it is important to know your full family history); starting menstrual periods at a young age (early menarche); ending periods at an older age (late menopause); and obesity. Risk factors do not cause breast cancer, but may contribute to its development. For example, the early onset of menstrual periods is not the cause of breast cancer, but it is thought that a longer time of ovarian cycling and estrogen production leads to more circulating estrogen over many years, which results in greater opportunity for breast cancer development.

A risk factor is anything that can contribute to the likelihood of getting breast cancer, but it is important to know the details that make someone more susceptible to breast cancer:

- **Age.** A woman's chance of developing breast cancer increases with age. Most occurrences of breast cancer happen in women older than fifty. By the time you are in your thirties, you may have a 1-in-233 chance of developing breast cancer. If you live to be eighty-five, your chance is 1-in-8.
- **A personal history of breast cancer.** If you have had breast cancer in one breast, you have an increased risk of developing breast cancer in the other breast.
- **Family history.** If you have an immediate family member—mother, sister, or daughter—with breast cancer or ovarian cancer or both, or even a male relative with breast cancer, you will have an increased risk of developing breast cancer in your lifetime. In theory, the more relatives you have that were diagnosed with breast cancer and were premenopausal when they contracted it, the higher your own risk will be. If you have one first-degree relative (mother, sister, daughter) who contracted the disease before the age of fifty or before menopause, then your chances of getting breast cancer doubles. If you have more relatives that have had breast cancer, then your odds of contracting breast cancer increase even more.
- **Obesity.** In general, studies indicate that there is a strong correlation between increased weight and breast cancer, especially for those with a weight increase in adolescence or after menopause. Body fat composition in the upper body also increases your risk.

- **Radiation exposure.** If you received excessive radiation exposure to your chest as a child or young adult, you will have an increased risk of getting breast cancer. And your risk increases if you had radiation to your breast area during your developmental years. For example, women who had radiation treatment to the chest for Hodgkin's disease in their teens have an increased risk of breast cancer.
- **First pregnancy at an older age.** If you have never been pregnant or you had your first pregnancy after the age of thirty, you have a greater chance of developing breast cancer. The theory is that pregnancy provides a mechanism that helps protect breast tissue from estrogen effects.
- **Race.** It is well documented that white women are more likely to get breast cancer. However, women of African American, Hispanic, or Asian descent are more likely to die of the disease. Studies have shown that these women are diagnosed when they are at a more advanced stage and have a more aggressive tumor. Socioeconomic factors, such as income, also influence the disparity of access to screening among different ethnic groups and affect the routine medical care that women in these groups receive or seek, according to studies.
- **Hormone therapy.** Treatment of postmenopausal symptoms with hormone therapy can increase the risk of breast cancer in those women who have taken hormone therapy for four or more years. The combination of estrogen and progesterone leads to greater risk than estrogen alone. Also, hormone therapy can increase breast density and make it harder to detect tumors on mammograms.
- **Birth control pills.** The role of oral contraceptives is controversial. Some studies say that the use of birth control pills for four or more years has been associated with an increased risk of breast cancer in premenopausal women. The risk is greater for those women who took birth control pills prior to

3

their first pregnancy. That risk may be partially because of delayed first pregnancy, which is also a risk factor.

- **Smoking.** There are varied theories about smoking and its link to breast cancer. Some studies show no risk and others suggest that there is a link to breast cancer risk. Overall, quitting smoking has great health benefits for all women.
- **Alcohol consumption.** There is controversy regarding the relationship of alcohol consumption to breast cancer risk. Some studies suggest that there is a 20 percent increased risk of breast cancer when women consume one or more alcoholic beverages a day, compared to women who do not drink. Other recent studies have indicated that red wine has some protective elements in lowering the risk of breast cancer. In general, it is recommended that a woman limit her consumption of alcoholic beverages to no more than one drink a day.
- **Presence of breast carcinoma in situ (e.g., LCIS) and other breast changes (e.g., atypical ductal hyperplasia).** These changes are usually discovered after a breast biopsy is performed because of an abnormal mammogram. Changes such as atypical hyperplasia or lobular carcinoma in situ increase one's risk of breast cancer. It is recommended that you develop a monitoring plan through discussion with your doctor and establish a follow-up plan that you are comfortable with.
- **Dense breasts.** The presence of dense breasts found with a mammogram indicates that there is a high ratio of connective and glandular tissue to fat. This makes it harder to detect masses or tumors with a mammogram. Having dense breasts is typically associated with premenopausal women with higher estrogen levels in the body, resulting in greater amounts of dense glandular tissue.

Fact

> In situ (Latin for "in its original place") breast carcinoma describes a type of precancerous cells that remain in one location and have not spread to surrounding tissue.

BRCA1 and BRCA2 Genes

You don't inherit cancer, but you can inherit an increased risk of developing cancer. There are now lab tests done on blood that can tell if you have inherited one of the abnormal high-risk breast cancer-related genes, BRCA1 or BRCA2. If you have such a gene, then your risk of developing breast cancer, particularly at a younger age, is much higher than normal.

If on one side of the family (father's or mother's) there are multiple women with breast cancer, women with breast cancer onset younger than age fifty, or women who have both ovarian cancer and breast cancer, then there is concern about the family having a BRCA1 or BRCA2 gene. Just because you have two or more relatives with breast or ovarian cancer does not mean that you have the hereditary form of breast cancer. Most women with a strong family history of breast cancer and who are at risk for the disease do not have the inherited breast cancer gene. Only about 5 percent of women with breast cancer have the inherited BRCA1 or BRCA2 genes.

The Role of the Immune System in Cell Growth and Metastasis

Bernard Fisher—a giant in breast cancer treatment research—recognized the possibility of breast cancer being a systemic disease even if seemingly localized to the breast. He promoted the idea of removing the axillary lymph nodes as a diagnostic or staging procedure rather than purely a treatment procedure. Fisher's research led to how people today look at breast cancer treatment and the complexity of breast cancer growth patterns and predictors of whether the cancer will spread.

 Fact

Metastasis is the migration of cancer cells to other organs. Those organs will become damaged if the cancer is not effectively treated.

Breast cancer can spread to lungs, liver, bones, and other parts of the body. Diagnosis tests are done to help assess the likelihood that the cancer is metastatic, meaning it will likely spread. Examination of lymph nodes will often be done, and in patients with more advanced cancer, such as those with multiple positive nodes or skin involvement, bone and CT scans may be done to look for metastatic disease. If any of the tests are positive for metastasis in areas outside the breast and axillary nodes, then the physician will often recommend systemic chemotherapy or hormonal therapy such as tamoxifen.

What to Expect—a Basic Timeframe

A timeframe for what to expect after first being diagnosed with breast cancer, and all the events that evolve from the initial diagnosis to the treatment phase, varies from individual to individual, but the main elements are similar. The following steps demonstrate a framework of the basic steps and timeframe:

1. Abnormality found on mammogram or abnormality found in clinical exam from self-breast exam or by your clinician
2. Doctor visit and examination
3. Radiological imaging tests (ultrasound, MRI) that may be indicated depending on the abnormal findings

4. If imaging result indicates a suspicious area, a breast biopsy will be done to further evaluate it. The type of biopsy varies (see Chapter 3). If the lump can be felt, a biopsy can be done in an office setting. If the lump cannot be felt, a mammogram-directed technique called stereotactic needle biopsy may be used. In this procedure, an ultrasound or mammogram is used to guide the needle for the biopsy. The choice of whether it will be a mammogram-directed stereotactic biopsy or an ultrasound-directed one depends on the type and location of the suspicious area, as well as the preference and the experience of the doctor. Some patients need a surgical excisional biopsy, in which the surgeon removes the lump or suspicious area along with normal-appearing breast tissue, called a margin.

5. A breast biopsy and examination under a microscope, which may take several days, will determine whether the suspicious area is positive for breast cancer. You may ask for a copy of your pathology report after a careful explanation of the report has been given to you by a doctor.

6. After breast cancer has been diagnosed, other tests are used to determine if the cancer has spread and to help determine the best treatment. These tests include chest x-ray, bone scan, CT or CAT scans, MRI, blood tests, complete blood counts (CBC), tumor tests for estrogen and progesterone receptor status, HER-2, breast cancer grade, and stage of breast cancer.

7. A determination may be made as to whether the patient is eligible for clinical trials.

It can take several weeks to a month from the time of the initial discovery and the breast cancer diagnosis, until the specifics of your breast cancer can be determined and a treatment plan that is best for you can be decided by your doctor and yourself.

Think about Your Treatment

The most crucial time in the process comes once you have been diagnosed with breast cancer and your treatment options have been presented in a way that you understand. It is now time to collect all your information and seek opinions from your medical team. Whatever the options that are presented, you need to sit back and process the steps involved and what impact it will have on you. Surgery may be recommended first, or chemotherapy may be advised prior to surgery, usually to shrink the tumor. In recent years there has also been increased use of preoperative chemotherapy, particularly for larger cancers.

 Alert

Remember, this is new territory for you and it may be the first time you have had to deal with a serious illness. Learning about your breast cancer is a slow process, which is a good thing. It takes time to sort through all the information that is given to you as well as time to adjust to the new life on which you are about to embark.

Today there are many options for women. Which direction you go in is often a personal choice that you make in concert with the advice and counsel of your doctor. Treatment now varies from conservation treatment which saves the breast—such as a lumpectomy and node biopsy—to a total bilateral mastectomy as a preventative measure for those who carry the breast cancer gene. This gene predisposes a woman to developing breast cancer and some might choose this treatment to decrease their chances of developing breast cancer in their lifetime.

Surgical removal and radiation are directed at the cancer in the breast and axillary nodes. Medicines such as chemotherapy, endocrine treatment, and antibodies may be used to treat cancer that has spread outside the breast region. Research suggests that complementary therapies such as meditation, yoga, positive thinking, and visualization are some of the treatments that may improve overall quality of life in women with breast cancer. Other research is being done to see if such practices also influence the biology and outcomes of cancer. This will be further discussed in Chapter 11. Most often, these complementary therapies are used together with traditional therapies, such as systemic chemotherapy, hormonal therapy, and radiation treatment.

Understand the sequence of treatment that will be needed and be careful not to jump into one treatment mode—think through the progression. For example, if you are considering a mastectomy with reconstruction at a later date, and you have had radiation to that breast, it will have a significant impact on your reconstructive surgery options.

 Fact

On average, it takes 100 days or more for a cancer cell to double in size. It takes about 10 years for cells to divide to a size that can be actually felt. So in a strict medical sense, it is not the dire emergency that you think it is. However, from an emotional perspective, one tends to think only about getting the cancer out and treating it so that it will not reoccur.

Too often women rush to decisions about treatment without doing the necessary homework that would allow them to make good choices. If you are diagnosed with breast cancer, it is important to slow down and get the right information so you can make those good choices. There is no data to suggest that quick surgery or other treatment is needed. The tumor has been growing for years and a few weeks here or there will not make a difference. Too much emotion can cloud decisions that you will have to live with for many years.

CHAPTER 2

What Does Breast Cancer Mean?

A fter your diagnosis, you will be bombarded with medical information. Trying to make sense of it while you are too upset to even think of treatment in a rational way is difficult. This chapter will explain breast cancer and some of the medical information that is given to you during the initial diagnosis. The more you learn, the more you realize that breast cancer is not just one diagnosis with one treatment choice, and you also can't compare one breast cancer situation to another. This chapter touches on the key elements that help you and your doctor make treatment choices. Knowledge is power and with that power comes the ability to make better treatment decisions.

Types of Breast Cancer

Once you have received a diagnosis of breast cancer, you want to know what type of breast cancer you have. There are many different types of cancer and each is named for the part of the breast the cancer most resembles. Current thinking suggests that both lobular and ductal tumors start in ductal tissue, but that lobular tumors start in the smaller terminal lobules. Their names reflect what the cancers look like. Most breast cancer (more than 80 percent) is ductal, appearing with glandular or ductal features under the microscope. Breast cancer that looks more like lobular tissue makes up about 12 percent of breast cancers and has single file invasive features. The remaining breast cancers include mucinous, medullary, papillary types, or are cancers of the tissue surrounding the ductal and lobular tissues.

 Question

What are ducts and lobules?
Ducts are tubes that carry milk to the nipple in the breast. The lobules are the glands that make the milk pass through the ducts.

Lobules and ducts are kinds of glands and the prefix *adeno* means "related to a gland." This is why breast cancer is referred to as an *adenocarcinoma*. Intraductal carcinoma or ductal carcinoma in situ (DCIS) is thought of as a precancer and is more contained within the duct. The cells look abnormal with cancerous features but have not invaded tissue outside the duct. That is, they are *in situ*, Latin for "in its original place."

Invasive or infiltrating ductal cancers tend to form a firm mass, often with associated fibrous tissue in the lump. Infiltrating lobular cancer is more insidious, because it sends individual cells out like tentacles into the surrounding tissue without a lot of reaction in that tissue and it can feel more like a thickening rather than a discrete firm mass. With lobular cancer, it is harder for the surgeon to know if it is all excised, because it can't be felt as easily as a hard lump. Lobular cancer has a higher tendency to occur in both breasts. Other types of breast cancer, including medullary, mucinous, and papillary breast cancers, each have their own microscopic patterns. The answer to which type of breast cancer you have can only be found out by your breast biopsy results, which will be further discussed in Chapter 3.

Tumor Size

The size of the tumor can be an important factor in choosing the appropriate treatment, especially with the use of adjuvant chemotherapy and breast conserving therapy with a lumpectomy. Size matters when it comes to breast cancer, but it is not everything. You can have a small tumor with an aggressive personality or a large tumor that is slow-growing and mild-mannered. Prediction of size prior to surgery is done primarily by imaging studies (i.e., mammography, ultrasound) and core biopsy. Clinical breast exam (CBE) by a physician or surgeon is not that reliable for predicting size. Recent studies indicate that ultrasound to detect tumor size is more accurate than other methods, such as CBE and mammography.

 Fact

Most tumors become visible on an x-ray when the diameter is 5mm to 10mm, but cannot be felt until they are about 10mm. The size of the tumor can only be accurately measured when it is surgically removed and examined by the pathologist. However, there is a lot of error in tumor measurement size because tumors are often irregular in shape. Different pathologists may come up with different sizes. This can be important, because often too much emphasis is placed on a few millimeters of size.

In one study, "Modeling the Effect of Tumor Size in Early Breast Cancer," the authors looked at the relationship between tumor size and mortality in early stage breast cancer. The data was taken from women diagnosed with breast cancer from 1988–1997 who presented with early stage breast cancer and had axillary node dissections and no metastasis. The conclusions of this study indicated that, regardless of node status, mortality increased with the size of the tumor from 10 percent to 25 percent for node-negative women (no cancer cells in the lymph nodes) to 20 percent to 40 percent for node-positive women.

Tumor growth seems to vary greatly between tumors, with faster growth rates found more often among younger women. Early detection among women will affect the size of the tumor found upon diagnosis and hopefully have an impact on overall mortality. However it is important to remember that it is not just size, but rather the tumor biology, that determines the likelihood of the cancer metastasizing to other parts of the body. Even with early detection, some cancers will behave badly. Unfortunately many primary care doctors and radiologists are threatened with lawsuits for so-called "late" or "missed" diagnoses of breast cancer. These suits are very often based on poor understanding of cancer biology. This threatening climate can cloud thinking about how cancer behaves and might lead to over-testing.

Tumor Grade

Once the type of cancer is determined, the pathologist (a doctor who studies the biology of tumors), will look further into the cells to determine the grade of the tumor. The grade of the tumor is an indication of how aggressively the cells might behave. Pathologists grade the tumors from 1 to 3, with the higher number being the worst prognosis. They also look to see if there are cells in the middle of a blood vessel or lymph vessel. This helps them determine how well behaved a cell is in the tissue. The pathologist looks at the margins of the tissue by putting ink around the outside of the sample, so she can measure the amount of normal tissue between the edge of the specimen and the cancer tissue. This is called the tumor margin.

If cancer is only on the inside and not beyond the ink drawn by the pathologist, then it is referred to as having a clear margin or a negative margin (a sign that no obvious cancer was left behind in that area). A positive margin means that cancer cells are found at the outer edge of the removed sample and is usually a sign that some cancer may still be present in the body. This still is an educated guess and the doctors can't be 100 percent sure. When there are questions, seeking a second opinion is advised.

 Question

What is a breast cancer margin?
A margin is the amount of normal tissue between the edge of a cancerous area and the cut surface of the sample or lump removed during surgery. Larger margins are better. Close or positive margins are associated with more cancer recurrence near the area of the tumor.

Lymph Node Status

Lymph nodes are bean-shaped glands under a woman's armpit or axilla that are part of the body's lymphatic system. The lymphatic system is a series of lymph glands that deliver lymphocytes (cells that fight infections found in the lymph fluid) to other parts of the body. Lymph nodes are an important part of the body's immune system that wards off infection. When lymph nodes contain breast cancer cells, the cancer is considered to be node positive. When the lymph nodes are clear of cancer cells then they are said to be negative. To determine if there are any cancer cells in the lymph nodes, the doctor will examine a sample from the lymph nodes under a microscope.

There are two tests that are used to indicate node status: the sentinel lymph node biopsy and the axillary lymph node dissection. The sentinel lymph node biopsy is a newer and now-routine procedure that usually involves injecting both a blue dye and a radioisotope into the central part of the breast. These materials will drain from the breast to a lymph node in the axilla. The first node reached is called the "sentinel" node. Using a Geiger counter–type device, the isotope is identified and the surgeon can see the blue dye. This allows the sentinel node to be removed for examination. If the sentinel node is negative, then it is assumed with a fair amount of accuracy that the rest of the nodes will be negative as well, and the woman is spared from having a large amount of lymph node tissue removed as it is in a routine axillary node dissection.

If the sentinel lymph node is positive, then a full node dissection is usually done with the added risk of possible chronic arm edema. With axillary node dissection, the risk of serious arm swelling (lymphedema) increases because the lymphatic system, which helps with natural fluid circulation and drainage in the upper arms and extremities, is disturbed. The sentinel lymph node procedure is minimally painful. Medication is given before the procedure and anti-anxiety medication can also be given if the patient and her doctor feel that it is necessary. Axillary lymph node dissections are more involved and usually done under general anesthesia.

 In Her Own Words

I have a large swollen arm from my fingertips to my armpit. Total strangers come up to me and ask, "What is wrong with your arm?" My five year-old granddaughter asks if Grandma's arm will ever get small. Mine is from the radiation to the lymph nodes in my armpit. I have to wear compression sleeves—one during the day and another at night. I have to use a pump with my arm in a sleeve to reduce the swelling. I have gotten infections, cellulitis, from bug bites and from no reason at all, and had to go to the hospital for intravenous antibiotics. I can't go in hot tubs. I can't get cuticles clipped on that hand or have my blood pressure measured, or shots in that arm. Lymphedema is a nuisance, but considering the alternatives, I am a very thankful woman.

—Marian, age 68, 15-year survivor

Lymph node involvement indicates how aggressive the tumor is. Previously, lymph node dissections were routinely done during breast cancer surgery and a large sample of nodes were examined individually to see if any cells were present. Lymph node involvement is thought of in terms of three types: minimal (microscopic), which has one to three-node involvement; significant (macroscopic), which has involvement of four to nine nodes; and extra-capsular extension, in which the tumor takes over the entire node and goes outside the wall of the lymph node and into the surrounding tissue. Doctors use the following categories to categorize lymph node involvement:

- No lymph nodes involved
- One to three nodes involved
- Four to nine nodes involved
- Ten or more nodes

It is thought that the more lymph nodes involved, the greater the risk that the cancer has spread to distant organs (metastasized). The specific involvement in each node is not as important as the total number of lymph nodes involved. More recently, the sentinel node biopsy is done before a full node dissection and since most breast cancers are node-negative, many women are spared the more involved procedure.

Lymphedema

Lymphedema is an abnormal swelling that occurs when there is a blockage in the lymphatic system, which then cannot adequately drain the circulating lymph fluid. This swelling can be caused in the arms and legs by a tumor or cancer cells blocking the lymph vessels, or can occur in the arms as a result of lymph node removal as part of cancer surgery, because of damage from radiation therapy, or because of injury or infection in the lymph node area.

In addition to the discomfort and cosmetic effects, the swollen arm is at greater risk for serious infection from even minor injuries, such as finger cuts.

Question

What is lymphedema?
Lymphedema is swelling caused by a collection of excess lymph fluid, brought about by a blockage in the lymphatic system. This complication may happen after the axillary lymph nodes (under the armpits) are removed during surgery, or are injured during radiation therapy. It may also be caused by a tumor interfering with the normal drainage of fluid. Lymphedema can be permanent after breast surgery and can be very difficult to manage, even with vigorous massage and exercise. The best management is prevention, which is why the sentinel node procedure is one of the most important breast cancer advances in recent years.

There is no cure for lymphedema, but the symptoms can be eased with diligent care of the limb or limbs that are affected. The symptoms may include severe fatigue, a heavy swollen limb, or localized fluid accumulation in the limb. Pain with the uncomfortable weight or fluid retention can also add to lymphedema problems. Treatments focus on minimizing the swelling and controlling the pain. Lymphedema treatments include:

- **Therapeutic exercise.** Light exercise may be recommended by a lymphedema therapist or physical therapist to help with lymph fluid drainage. These exercises are not to cause fatigue but to enhance circulation and promote a gentle contraction of the muscles in the arms to help keep the tissue soft and assist in moving the lymphedema fluid. The exercises should be prescribed in consultation with a physician to promote function and comfort during the patient's treatments.
- **Manual lymph drainage/decongestive therapy.** This is a known tool for lymphedema management that involves manual manipulation of the lymphatic ducts for the purpose of encouraging lymph flow away from the affected arm and

back to healthy lymph nodes where the excess fluid can drain. The technique was founded by Emil Vodder in the 1930s for the treatment of immune disorders and sinusitis. Manual lymph drainage involves gentle, rhythmic massaging of the skin to stimulate flow of the lymphatic system and reduce swelling. A session usually lasts forty to sixty minutes and manipulation of the skin starts with the neck, trunk, and then the affected limb.

- **Compression wrapping or bandaging.** Compression wrapping, in which the entire arm is wrapped, helps with encouraging lymph fluid to drain from the extremity toward the trunk of the body. When bandaging your arm, you need to wrap tighter at the end of your limbs and loosen it as you go up toward the body. This helps to facilitate lymphatic flow by providing a pump-like pressure going from the fingers toward the body. It is advised to use short-stretch bandages as opposed to the long-stretch bandages used to treat sprains, because the short-stretch bandages encourage lymphatic flow and help to soften swollen tissue. This must be first taught by a physical therapist or lymphedema specialist with ongoing follow-up and monitoring. Proper placement of compression wrapping is essential in promoting proper lymph drainage.

- **Compression garments.** These include long sleeves worn by the person with lymphedema following decongestive therapy to reduce and minimize edema. Compression garments are worn to reduce swelling and usually need to be worn every day and must be replaced on a regular basis. Depending on the recommendation of the therapist, the patient may have an over-the-counter standard size or may have to have a custom-fit compression garment. Currently there is controversy about compression sleeves. Some today would argue that decongestive massage techniques and specialized

wraps are better than the older style sleeves. It is often difficult to get insurance coverage for lymphedema treatments
and compression garments, so you may need to check with
your local breast cancer center for available resources in
your area.

- **Pneumatic compression.** In this treatement, a compression
pump moves the lymph fluid gently with a pneumatic sleeve
attached to the pump. This is usually done for ten to fifteen
minutes prior to manual lymph drainage. The pump sequen-
tially inflates and deflates the sleeve in order to move lymph
fluid away from your fingers and toward your body to help
recirculate the excess fluid and reduce swelling.

- **Skin care.** People with lymphedema or whose lymph nodes
have been removed are at higher risk for infections in the
affected areas. Special care of your skin with gentle cleansing and moisturizing is important to promote circulation of
lymph fluid and prevent cuts or other damage to the skin
that could result in a skin infection of the affected area.

Lymphedema Prevention and Coping

All women with lymph node dissections or radiation to the
axilla or supraclavicular areas are at risk for lymphedema. To
reduce your risk of lymphedema you can:

- Keep your skin clean, and protect your arm and breast area
from injury. Avoid skin tears or cuts that may contribute to
the possibility of an infection. Wear a glove when gardening
or doing other tasks where skin injury may occur.

- Elevate your arm on a pillow at night or whenever possible
after your breast surgery.

- Avoid tight or constricting clothing that may hinder circulation in the affected arm. Avoid carrying a bag over the shoulder on the side of the node dissection. After a node operation,

much of the lymph returns to the body through lymphatics over the shoulder, and a purse or other strapped bag can cut off that circulation.

Find out all you can about lymphedema so that you understand its causes and symptoms. This information will help guide you when you make decisions about your treatment options. The more you know, the better able you will be to facilitate your treatment and speak to your doctor and physical therapist about what you are experiencing. This type of conversation will help them plan your individual treatment strategy.

Take good care of your affected arm by gentle cleansing and taking safety precautions to avoid injury to the affected limb from cuts or scratches. Be hypervigilant in caring for your skin by applying moisturizer daily to prevent dry skin and cracking.

Find other women who have experienced lymphedema in your area for support, or inquire about a lymphedema support group in your area. You can also contact the National Lymphedema Network, which may be able to refer you to others who have been through it and put you in contact with them. It is helpful to talk to others who have had this problem, because they can offer the help and support that only comes from experience.

Essential

Tumors have a biology of their own, and great strides have been made toward understanding cancer biology and how to manipulate it. Once you understand the tumor's biology, then you and your doctor can guide your treatment decisions. Staging breast cancer gives guidelines for comparison, so doctors can standardize diagnosis and treatment and understand outcomes in a way that is universal for patients and clinical centers.

Stages of Breast Cancer

The stage of your cancer is based on: the size of the tumor, whether the cancer is invasive or noninvasive, whether lymph nodes are involved, and whether it has spread beyond the breast and nodes. When you are going through this phase of your diagnosis, it is important to remember that information about your cancer comes at different times and this period can be the most stressful time of the cancer experience. Things settle down once you have the complete picture of your cancer, know what the size of the tumor is, what stage it's in, whether it is invasive or not, and whether your lymph nodes are involved. Then you can move forward in your treatment.

- **Stage 0.** Stage 0 means that there is no invasion of the cancer cells into the surrounding tissue. DCIS and LCIS are examples of Stage 0.
- **Stage I.** Stage I describes invasive breast cancer, in which the cells are breaking through to surrounding tissue and:
  - The tumor is 2 centimeters or less in greatest dimension AND
  - No lymph nodes are involved.
- **Stage II.** Stage II is divided into subgroups known as IIA and IIB.
  Stage IIA describes invasive breast cancer in which:
  - No tumor is found in the breast, but cancer cells are found in the axillary lymph nodes (lymph nodes under the arm), OR
  - The tumor measures 2 centimeters or less and has spread to the axillary lymph nodes, OR
  - The tumor is larger than 2 centimeters but less than 5 centimeters and has not spread to the axillary lymph nodes.

Stage IIB describes invasive breast cancer in which:
- The tumor is larger than 2 but less than 5 centimeters and has spread to the axillary lymph nodes, OR
- The tumor is larger than 5 centimeters but has not spread to the axillary lymph nodes.
- **Stage III.** Stage III is divided into subcategories known as IIIA, IIIB, and IIIC.

Stage IIIA describes invasive breast cancer in which either:
- No tumor is found in the breast. Cancer is found in the axillary nodes that are clumped together or sticking to other structures or the cancer has spread to the axillary nodes near the breastbone, OR
- The tumor is 5 centimeters or smaller and has spread to axillary lymph nodes that are clumped together or sticking to other structures, OR
- The tumor is larger than 5 centimeters and has spread to axillary lymph nodes that are clumped together or sticking to other structures.

Stage IIIB describes invasive breast cancer in which:
- The tumor may be any size and has spread to the chest wall and/or skin of the breast, AND
- The tumor may have spread to axillary lymph nodes that are clumped together or sticking to other structures or cancer may have spread to lymph nodes near the breastbone.

Stage IIIC describes invasive breast cancer in which:
- There may be no sign of cancer in the breast or, if there is a tumor, it may be any size and may have spread to the chest wall and/or skin of the breast, AND
- The cancer has spread to lymph nodes above or below the collarbone, AND
- The cancer may have spread to axillary lymph nodes or to lymph nodes near the breastbone.

- **Stage IV.** Stage IV describes invasive breast cancer that has spread to other organs of the body, usually the lungs, liver, bone, or brain. Stage IV breast cancer is called metastatic breast cancer.

It is important to remember that women often confuse *stage* and *grade*. If you review your pathology report, don't confuse grade (the pathologist's description of the cancer) with stage (the anatomic extent of the cancer).

Symptoms that occur in metastatic breast cancer relate to the organ that is affected. With metastasis to the lung, it is common to experience shortness of breath, or bone pain, which may indicate possible metastasis to the bones. Loss of appetite and weight loss suggest metastasis to the liver. It is important to note that the symptoms alone do not indicate metastasis, but will lead to additional testing to confirm the possibility of breast cancer metastasis to that organ. If you have Stage IV breast cancer, people will often treat you as if you are near death, often diminishing any hope and the pursuit of breast cancer treatment. A recent study indicated that 20 percent of women with metastatic breast cancer live five years or longer. The study also recognized that each breast cancer is unique and varies in its course of action. Many drugs are being developed and used for metastatic breast cancer treatment. It is always helpful to see yourself on the positive side of breast cancer survival, no matter what the statistics are.

Estrogen Receptor Status

Estrogen is a key player in the biology of breast cancer. Estrogen links with the estrogen receptor protein to influence breast tissue function. Estrogen receptor (ER) can be measured in the breast cancer tissue. It is one of the key bio-markers that is tested to help determine your course of treatment. Progesterone receptor (PR) is also an important test to perform on any breast cancer. A cancer that measures positive for either estrogen or progesterone or both receptors is considered hormone-receptor positive. Hormone receptors are like antennae on a cell. Estrogen sends signals through the receptors to tell breast cancer to grow. After a breast cancer is removed, the cancer cells are tested for estrogen and progesterone receptors. The more estrogen and progesterone receptors that are present, the more likely the cancer will respond to hormonal therapy. If the tumor does not have estrogen or progesterone receptors, antiestrogen therapy will not be helpful.

What this means is that the oncologist is looking to see if the tumor cells are likely to respond to anti-estrogen treatment. In general, tumors in postmenopausal women are more likely to be estrogen-receptor positive and tumors in premenopausal women estrogen-receptor negative. Knowing the receptor status helps to determine whether hormone replacement therapy is an option.

The S-phase lab test reveals the number of cells dividing in the tumor, the S-phase fraction usually showing how quickly a cell is dividing. A low S-phase fraction is an indication that the tumor is slow growing and a high S-phase fraction shows that the cells are rapidly dividing and that the tumor is more aggressive. This test is not available everywhere and gives the same information as nuclear grade, but is more reliable.

Biomarkers

Biomarkers are any trait of a tumor that can be tested to help categorize or assess the tumor. Tests for the presence of hormone receptors, and the amplification of certain genes such as HER-2, can help predict how the tumor might behave with and without treatment. Biomarkers can guide treatment decisions and options for care. For example a tumor that shows amplification (too many copies) of the gene HER-2 is more likely to respond to the antibody trastuzumab. This is one of the most successful biomarkers in breast cancer treatment today. Cell function is extremely complex and targeted breast cancer treatment refers to treatments that are directed at specific parts of the cell machinery such as the HER-2 dependent or the estrogen dependent pathways. Major efforts are underway to learn more about the details of how cancer cells turn on and off so that targets can be identified for possible treatment development.

If the doctor refers to your cancer as a triple negative tumor, it means that you have an estrogen- and progesterone- receptor-negative tumor and also a HER-2 negative tumor. In other words, your tumor is not going to benefit from hormone treatments or trastuzumab (Herceptin). With fewer tools to use as treatment, these cancers at present have only cytotoxic chemotherapy as possible systemic treatment options.

CHAPTER 3

Tests to Diagnose Breast Cancer

The world of medical diagnostic testing for breast cancer changes as new research and studies unfold. Currently, the primary tests used in the diagnosis of breast cancer include the imaging techniques of mammography (digital or film), MRI, ultrasound, and several breast biopsy methods. Traditional mammography is still the most widely used first choice for diagnostic testing; however it brings with it fear of uncertainty as well as discomfort. The drawbacks often cause women to postpone regular yearly mammograms, and that, in turn, contributes to delayed detection of breast cancer. The goal should always be early detection of breast cancer, because studies have shown that survival increases when breast cancer is detected in its early stages.

Traditional Mammography

A mammogram, or x-ray of the breast, is a method of detecting breast cancer tumors that cannot be felt. Mammograms are done with a special type of x-ray machine used only for mammograms and which produce a picture of the breast on film. There are two types of mammography: screening and diagnostic. Screening mammography is recommended annually after age forty and is used as a detection tool when there are no symptoms. The pictures are reviewed by a radiologist with methodical comparison to previous mammograms. Diagnostic mammography is the same detection tool, but is done when there's a problem, such as when a suspicious area in the breast needs further investigation. A lump that can be felt, or an abnormality seen on a screening mammogram, would spur a diagnostic mammogram.

In a mammogram, the breast is sandwiched between two plastic x-ray plates. It can be uncomfortable and pain can vary among individuals, depending on breast sensitivity. The actual time it takes to have a mammogram is three to five minutes and the actual compression time is about thirty seconds. The compression is done to spread out the tissue, which provides the best image to help to detect any abnormalities. During a mammogram, the x-ray is taken from two views, one from top to bottom and the other from side to side.

Mammograms highlight different densities in the breast tissue. The radiologist is skilled in interpreting the patterns he sees and is trained to identify changes that might be cancer.

Essential

Mammograms are far from perfect. Many abnormalities are labeled as possibly being cancer or are abnormal enough that a biopsy needs to be done. Some changes that can be confused with cancer include fibrocystic change, benign calcifications, or other normal breast densities.

Breast cancers have their own unique pattern. On an x-ray they appear irregularly shaped and often the edges radiate out like sun rays, called spiculations. About half of breast cancers show calcium deposits, which are also referred to as microcalcifications. Calcium deposits may normally appear in the breast and are often noncancerous and, depending on the size, shape, and appearance, will determine whether they are suspicious for breast cancer or not. In general microcalcifications that are clustered in a certain area of the breast and irregular in shape will warrant further investigation by a needle biopsy, which will be discussed later in this chapter.

A diagnostic mammogram is performed when there is a problem with the findings or questions regarding certain areas of the breast that are not well visualized. They include repeat views, additional views, or magnification views to look at a specific area.

Once you have been treated for breast cancer, you can expect to have repeat mammograms generally at least every twelve months. The exact schedule will vary with the institution. Women who have had a mastectomy will only have a mammogram on the remaining breast.

 Alert

Your first mammogram after breast cancer treatment will feel much different. You can be sure that the affected breast will be more tender and sore. Radiation and surgery will create changes within the breast resulting in pain, inflammation, and sensitivity of the breast tissue. This may lessen with time, but usually some increased sensitivity and discomfort will be experienced.

You may want to consider taking an anti-inflammatory (such as acetaminophen or ibuprofen) prior to going for your first posttreatment mammogram, but it is always recommended that you consult your doctor first.

Digital Mammography

Digital mammography does not use film, but rather stores the images electronically in a computer. This allows greater ability to manipulate the images; for instance, magnifying an area of interest. It also provides a more efficient system for moving the information electronically. This can be combined with a computer-aided detection (CAD) program (as can film mammography) and helps the radiologists to further interpret the findings.

Digital mammography offers a clearer image of the breast than traditional mammography in women with dense breast tissue. First-time digital mammography results may alarm some women, because often the radiologist has to call back for a repeat digital mammogram. The call back may occur because the radiologist cannot compare your first digital mammogram to your previous traditional mammogram. Don't be alarmed about a call back. It is important to remember that the radiologist is being diligent and that it is worth the extra step for peace of mind. Keep in mind that you need to feel comfortable with what is being presented to you, so ask the questions necessary to understand the information and help you to agree with the follow-up plan, whether it is careful watching or further investigation.

Digital mammography feels the same as standard mammography as far as breast compression and the overall procedure. The time needed to position a woman for the test is also the same. Digital mammography requires less than a minute to develop, whereas a standard mammogram requires several minutes to develop. Digital mammography provides a three-dimensional view of the breast, whereas standard mammography provides a two-dimensional image. However, currently only special units are equipped for 3D imaging. This will likely become standard in the future. Digital mammography is a computerized image that has a digital receptor and computer and stores its image on a computer instead of a film cassette. Digital mammography can also be enhanced and manipulated in order for the radiologist to see a clearer picture, especially in dense breasts, therefore detecting smaller lesions and making it possible to rule out noncancerous masses.

Ultrasound

Ultrasound is a sonogram method of diagnosis that uses a device called a transducer to generate high-frequency sound waves that are beamed through solid and fluid-filled structures of the body. No x-ray type radiation is involved with ultrasonography and it is a painless procedure. Normal body structures like the breast have varying types of tissues and structures and will absorb or reflect sound waves differently. This information is then transferred into a picture to be interpreted by the radiologist. Normal organs reveal certain ultrasound patterns while diseased organs have their own characteristic patterns. Newer machines can also show movement in "real time," which means that they can analyze motion as well as sound.

For an ultrasound, you generally will lie down on a table. The technician will place a gel on the area to block air between the transducer and the skin. Breast ultrasound is used for breast lumps because it can detect whether it is a fluid-filled cyst or a solid mass. Breast ultrasound is generally not used for screening, but it has recently been given some attention as a complement to mammography in certain situations.

Magnetic Resonance Imaging (MRI)

Magnetic resonance imaging, or MRI, is a breast-imaging technique that captures multiple cross-sectional pictures of your breast. Breast MRI consists of combining these images using a computer to generate detailed pictures, which are displayed on a monitor. It differs from x-rays in that MRI uses a large, powerful magnet to send magnetic waves through the body and then records the returning waves, making images appear on a computer screen. This is one of the newest high-tech tests and provides valuable images. You may not be able to have an MRI of the breast if you have any metal equipment or clips in your body, such as a pacemaker, ear implant, metal clips in your eyes, implanted port devices, an intrauterine device (IUD), metal plates, pins, screws, or surgical staples. Some implanted devices are made of material that will not be affected by the MRI. In recent years, staples and other objects have been made of non-ferromagnetic material and are safe with MRI. Be sure to tell your doctor if you have any metal objects in your body that may interfere with the MRI equipment and find out if those objects are safe or not.

An MRI is most effective in detecting smaller breast cancer tumors. MRIs are the most accurate diagnostic tool for the disease and can detect 79 percent to 98 percent of cancerous tumors. However, in some situations, the test is too sensitive and non-cancer changes are mistaken for cancer. This is a real problem when using MRI for screening. Because of the high cost, it is not as widely used a screening tool, but for women at high risk for developing breast cancer it may be recommended. A study in high-risk women indicated that tumors found by MRI combined with mammography were significantly smaller and less likely to have spread to the lymph nodes. It is also known that in younger women who have denser breasts, traditional mammography has its limitations, and therefore combining mammography with MRIs can be more effective.

Your doctor may order an MRI of your breast to evaluate breast abnormalities seen on a mammogram or for women with dense breast tissue, implants, or scar tissue that interferes with regular breast imaging with mammography. An MRI may also be used to evaluate the progress of your breast cancer treatment as well as identifying cysts, enlarged ducts, hematomas, or leaking or ruptured breast implants. In general, MRIs are not ordered for screening of benign and malignant tumors because of the high cost of the process and the fact the technology is so sensitive that it often mistakes non-cancer changes for cancer. You may advocate for an MRI of your breast by asking your doctor if it might be recommended for your situation. However if your doctor does not recommend it, be sure to understand her rationale for not indicating it for your situation.

What to Expect

Before your doctor schedules an MRI, she will likely do a physical exam and take a medical history, do a pregnancy test if you are premenopausal, assess any allergies you may have, and perhaps prescribe a mild sedative if you have anxiety or fear of enclosed places. Before your MRI, you may be asked to avoid using hairsprays, hair gel, lotions, and powders and cosmetics, because metallic substances used in some of these may interfere with the imaging. The best time to schedule an MRI is between days seven and fourteen of the menstrual cycle if you are premenopausal. If you take a mild sedative for this test, you should arrange for someone to drive you to and from the procedure.

Essential

Most MRI centers will have music available to help calm you during the procedure. The MRI machine makes loud noises during the procedure and your technician will alert you to this so that you have advance warning of the strange noises you may hear. Other relaxation techniques, such as meditation, centering practices of focusing on the breath, prayer, and yoga may be very helpful before your MRI.

Once you are at the MRI center, you will be asked to remove any metal objects, such as jewelry, watches, hearing aids, glasses, wigs, and nonpermanent dentures. There is no pain associated with the procedure, so you will not need any anesthesia. During your MRI, you lie face-down on your stomach in a movable bed. Your breasts will hang into cushioned openings, during which the bed slides into a large, cylindrical-shaped magnet. You may be hooked up to monitors to check your pulse and heart rate during the procedure. If your doctor has ordered an MRI with contrasting dye, then you will have a saline solution with contrast dye injected through an intravenous (IV) line into your hand or arm. The technician will leave the room during the procedure. The procedure without contrast dye takes about thirty to forty minutes and up to one and a half hours for an MRI with contrast dye.

Breast Biopsy

The type of breast cancer you have can only be discovered by a breast biopsy, in which tissue from the tumor is extracted and then tested in the lab. You need to understand what type of breast cancer you have before you can weigh your treatment options and make a decision. There are four breast biopsy procedures:

- Fine-needle aspiration
- Core biopsy
- Incisional biopsy
- Excisional biopsy

The first and least invasive is the fine-needle aspiration. This is usually done at the doctor's office, most often by a surgeon or other breast cancer specialist. During the fine-needle aspiration, the doctor holds the lump, gives local anesthetics to numb the tissue around the lump, and then passes the needle in and out a few times to get out cells that can be analyzed. This results in material that yields a cytology report, or an examination of a smear of cells.

The second type is a core biopsy, which consists of removing a core from the center of the suspicious mass using a needle device. This can also be done easily in the doctor's office. A core biopsy yields a greater amount of tissue than fine-needle aspiration.

In an incisional biopsy a wedge is taken out of the lump. This is done under local anesthetic. An incisional biopsy does not attempt to get good margins around the cancer and should rarely if ever be used for evaluation of a mass that is suspicious for cancer. If a lump is not palpated but is seen on mammography, it is done with guidance of wire localization with the abnormal area being marked with wires or needles under image guidance. The surgeon then follows the wire to get out the area that is localized. For an excisional biopsy, the surgeon takes out the whole lump.

Each type of breast biopsy has its pros and cons. The choice of which type is used depends on your particular situation. Your doctor will recommend one over another by evaluating how suspicious the tumor looks, how large it is, where it is in your breast, how many tumors are present, and your personal preference. Incisional biopsies are generally not ideal and in recent years a core biopsy has been the most common first step at getting tissue. You may want to discuss this with your doctor, understanding the rationale for choosing one biopsy over another. Remember, whenever medical information is presented to you, it is important that it makes sense to you, so that you will be comfortable with having the procedure.

QUESTIONS TO ASK YOUR DOCTOR WHEN YOU HAVE A BIOPSY SCHEDULED
1. What type of biopsy do you recommend? Why?
2. How soon will I know the results?
3. What will the biopsied area look like as it heals?
4. What type of anesthetic are you recommending, local or general anesthesia?
5. What are the pros and cons of local anesthesia? Of general anesthesia?

TIPS FOR DISCUSSING YOUR BIOPSY RESULTS WITH YOUR DOCTOR
1. Request a copy of your pathology report and ask your doctor to explain it to you.
2. Ask what type of breast cancer you have.

3. Ask if the estrogen-receptor status was tested on the tissue biopsy and what the results mean.
4. Ask if any other lab tests were done on your tissue sample and what the results mean.
5. Ask what the next steps are, whether you need additional testing, and why or why not.

Remember, if your instincts are telling you that something is wrong, be sure to pursue your concerns with your doctor. If you are not satisfied with the information you are given, seek a second and even a third opinion if you feel it is necessary.

Genetic Testing

Genetic testing, which involves analysis of your DNA, is still a debated issue in breast cancer treatment. Genetic testing for breast cancer tests for a genetic change or mutation also found in a number of other people who have contracted breast cancer.

If your family has a high incidence of breast or ovarian cancer, you may want to be tested for the gene changes that predispose you to breast cancer. In breast and ovarian cancer, the susceptible genes are called BRCA1 and BRCA2. If you have these genes with specific mutations, you have a significantly higher risk of getting these diseases.

In Her Own Words

After being diagnosed with breast cancer and speaking to my doctor about family history, it was a real wake-up call to actually see how many people, especially the women in my family, had either breast or ovarian cancer. Being tested for the BRCA gene has probably saved my life.

—Donna, age 52, 1-year survivor

Mutations of the BRCA1 and BRCA2 genes account for about 36 to 85 percent of the breast cancer that occurs in women with strong family histories of the disease. In other words, women with this gene mutation have a three to seven times higher risk than women without the gene. It is highest in families with a history of multiple cases of breast cancer, cases of both breast and ovarian cancer, and one or more family members with two primary cancers, such as the original tumor present in two different sites, or in those women of Ashkenazi Jewish background (Eastern Europe). Also, women with an inherited alteration in one of these genes have an increased risk of developing breast cancer at a younger age (before menopause).

 Alert

The fear of having your health insurance carrier discover the results of your test, especially if you have tested positive for the breast cancer gene, is a real concern with many women. Gene testing and its impact on health insurance coverage has received much publicity and lawmakers are working on changes that will protect against discrimination by insurance companies.

Before you decide to have genetic testing done, it is recommended that you seek genetic counseling. A genetic counselor or physician with interest in the area will help you look at your family and medical history and discuss in detail your risk of developing breast cancer. A genetic counselor can not only help you decide if you want to be tested, and what this means to you, but can also provide support before and after genetic testing. Although genetic testing is done with a simple blood test, it carries psychological, ethical, and social issues that need to be addressed to help with the decision-making process and the implications of what you do with the information in the future.

The lifetime risk of developing breast cancer in women found with the BRCA1 and BRCA2 mutated genes range is 40 percent to as high as 85 percent. There is also a 15 to 45 percent chance of developing ovarian cancer. Women who have the inherited mutations in BRCA1 or BRCA2 but have not been diagnosed with breast cancer may want to consider preventive strategies, such as prophylactic mastectomy (removing the breasts) or oophorectomy (removing the ovaries). Other women may choose "careful watching" by their doctor, with follow-up appointments every three months. Some women choose to use tamoxifen, an anti-estrogen hormone. Seriously consider whether or not to have genetic testing done, as the information this testing provides can influence your life in many ways.

 Fact

There is a new federal law that protects women from genetic discrimination. It is called the Genetic Information Nondiscrimination Act (GINA). The Coalition for Genetic Fairness has published an interactive online guide to GINA. You can access this guide online at *www .geneticfairness.org/ginaresource.html.*

A positive test result may have a direct impact on a person's emotions, relationships, finances, and medical choices. Genetic testing influences family members by revealing information about them, which may cause tension within families. Also some of those within the family that test negative may suffer from survivor guilt. Test results may also affect personal choices, such as marriage and decisions regarding having children.

The Waiting Game

Waiting for test results is the most stressful time in the breast cancer experience for many women. Knowing the results of all the combined tests shows you and your doctor the total picture of your breast cancer, which will guide your treatment options. It is recommended that you have a family member or friend with you when the doctor presents these options, so you have someone there who can help you process the information, take part in the discussion, and also to take notes.

When You'll Hear Results

At your first follow-up appointment after surgery, you usually will meet with your oncologist, who will be the doctor responsible for carrying out your breast cancer treatment post-surgery. In some cases, you may see the surgeon first, or you may meet with a team of medical experts to discuss options. For example, at a breast center, a team approach is often used. At this meeting you will find out the exact size of your tumor, the stage of your breast cancer, lymph node involvement, the estrogen-receptor status and HER-2 status of your breast cancer tumor, and other specifics, such as the S-phase, if tested. Ultimately, your treatment plan regarding chemotherapy and radiation after surgery will be a decision you make with the oncologist.

It may also be recommended by your doctor that you have chemotherapy before surgery (neoadjuvant chemotherapy, which is used for women with large, locally advanced breast cancer). Generally it is recommended that the tumor be shrunk before surgery to allow the surgeon the best possible chance of removing it. If the tumor shrinks considerably with chemotherapy, it can even change the surgical options from a mastectomy to a breast-conserving option. If you really want a breast-preservation approach but your doctor says the tumor is too big, you should at least ask about the possibility of preoperative chemotherapy. In some cases, but not all, this will shrink the tumor enough to allow a lumpectomy with good margins.

All of the specific characteristics of your breast tumor do not come to the doctor at the same time, but trickle in from the tumor's pathology report, blood tests, genetic testing (if done), the doctor's summary of, the whole picture, or consultation with another oncologist or breast cancer center before making a recommendation. Most hospitals have tumor rounds, in which breast cancer specialists, oncologists, surgeons, radiologists, pathologists, and other breast cancer professionals gather to discuss newly diagnosed breast cancer patients (in confidence, of course). They further interpret the tumor's results and the presenting symptoms of the patient or other information and each professional gives her input and perspective. This is a huge benefit to the patient—there are several doctors weighing in on your case and more is definitely better.

In Her Own Words

After getting re-mammogrammed on the left side, I was terrified, waiting in that little booth praying that all was well. The technician came back and said, "You can get dressed but the doctor wants to see you." I knew then that this was it. I was so afraid: Am I going to die? What am I going to do?

—Saundra, age 48, 1-year survivor

You can ask your oncologist if your case has been discussed during tumor rounds or can request that this be done, if available. These discussions do not take the place of a second opinion at a separate hospital or facility, but can provide additional information about your specific tumor. Having other specialists looking at your case objectively and making recommendations helps guide your treatment options, but it can also lend itself to more confusion if you don't understand everything that's being said. You should ask your doctor if there are any controversial issues in your case. If there are not, the doctor should make that clear. If there are, you should know what they are. This is why it is important to talk to your doctor with a family member or friend present. And remember, the information presented needs to make sense to you. You are embarking on a six- to twelve-month treatment plan and you want to make sure that you are comfortable with the treatment option you have chosen.

What to Expect Next

You can definitely count on the test results not coming back as fast as you would like. The waiting period for your test results will seem like an eternity. You want immediate confirmation and results and it will appear as if no one is on your timetable. Some tests are invasive and may cause pain, while others are non-invasive and may only require a blood draw, x-ray, or ultrasound. However, every test, whether it is arduous or not, causes anxiety. The emotional impact weighs heavily on the woman experiencing the test, even though the medical perception is that these tests are, for the most part, routine procedures.

Getting test results can be stress-provoking, and becomes your only focus until you finally have them. Whether you accept this process quietly and stoically or request medication to assist you in relieving the anxiety as you try to cope with the waiting period, it is difficult to go through this process. Solicit support from your anxious family and friends, but be assured that there is no good way to wait. One of the most trying times in the cancer journey is waiting for the initial test results.

Advocate for getting your results as soon as possible from your doctor, but know that there are often delays in getting these results because of your breast center's protocols on who can give you the information. You may receive your results from your oncologist, surgeon, or primary care doctor. The best person to find the results out from is the doctor you have a relationship with and to whom you can communicate your concerns and who can help you understand your test results. Many results can also be given by a knowledgeable breast cancer nurse.

CHAPTER 4

Exploring Your Options

O ptions seem to overwhelm you when you are first diagnosed with breast cancer. And it will become clear to you that breast cancer treatment is not an exact science. The process of exploring your options is slow and requires emotional as well as physical energy. This chapter will cover the factors that initially are overwhelming and can make the decision process more complex. It will discuss the feelings, emotions, and turmoil that will visit you as the exploring stage is filled with new information and new territory for you and your family. The goal of this chapter is to give you some tips that will help you make your treatment decision and arm you with information so you can partner with your doctor from a position of strength.

How to Choose Your Physician

The first and most important decisions you will make are choosing your medical oncologist, and also your surgeon. If you are having surgery, your surgeon is also part of this stage. To begin the process, ask your family doctor or your primary care doctor for a referral, especially if you have had a long relationship with him. Then share with your oncologist your medical history and what is important to you, your fears and concerns, and any personal factors that will have an impact on your treatment decisions. This will help you and your doctor review your options for treatment and decide on the treatment that best suits you.

This is one time that you do not need to be concerned about hurting anyone's feelings. It's okay to meet with two surgeons or oncologists and decide that you are more comfortable with one than the other. For example, as you go along this process, you learn of a physician in a nearby community, perhaps two hours away, who is considered an expert in the field of breast cancer and you want to see what this doctor can offer you as far as your breast cancer treatment. So you must be prepared to consider factors such as traveling to receive treatment, personal lifestyle, and family responsibilities when choosing your oncologist. These factors may sway you to receive local treatment or you may find that receiving breast cancer treatment from the doctor far from your home is better suited to your needs.

In Her Own Words

Luckily, all my doctors and nurses and the entire staff have been extremely approachable. I had to stress to my doctors that I have a needle phobia. Don't be afraid to share, the more you tell them, the more they can work with you. One-on-one conversations are the best way to communicate, and luckily, all of my doctors were kind enough to make that time for me. I also stress that bringing a friend/family with you when you meet with your doctor is key. There is so much information; it is difficult for one person to collect it all. Take lots of notes and save them.

—Pat, age 49, 6-month survivor

If you treat your doctor as your partner, it helps empower you as you seek information about your options for care. You may want to only understand the basics or you may choose to become well-versed in breast cancer treatment. However, try not to become an expert in the field by yourself, guided only by your own principles.

Whichever approach you choose, it is important that you are comfortable with your doctor and that he supports your decisions. In other words, choose a doctor who matches your needs and philosophy of care. For example, if you are a believer in complementary therapies and are an active participant in yoga practices, it may be important for you to incorporate this into your treatment plan. When searching for a doctor for your breast cancer treatment, you may ask if he is a proponent of your personal practice of yoga or if he has a strong opinion about it or any similar forms of complementary therapies. You make want to make your oncologist decision according to how important something like that is to you.

Once you have decided on your doctor, it is a good idea to ask if he would like to take you on as a new patient. This starts the process of open communication with your doctor that will build your future relationship and gives the doctor an opportunity to express his concerns about your breast cancer treatment decisions. Establishing open communication early on in your treatment will set you and your doctor up for a win-win situation.

Learn as Much as You Can about Your Choices and Challenges

The more you learn about the specifics of your breast cancer diagnosis, the better informed decision you will make. As discussed in the previous chapters, the size, stage, lymph node involvement, HER-2 status, and estrogen receptor status will assist you in choosing, along with your doctor, your best breast cancer treatment. It is your right and responsibility to understand the information that has been presented to you.

The dilemma is that there is no one right decision or choice in your breast cancer treatment. The more information you have about your specific breast cancer—its characteristics, size, and so on—the more confident in your decision you will be. This is the time that you should not leave any stone unturned as far as the information available to you.

Once you have had all the necessary diagnostic tests and biopsies, the next step is to decide on your treatment of choice, whether you will have a full mastectomy of the affected breast, bilateral prophylactic mastectomy, lumpectomy and radiation, lumpectomy with radiation and chemotherapy, or lumpectomy and adjuvant chemotherapy (adjuvent therapy is a treatment that aids the effectiveness of the primary treatment). There are other choices for older women, such as whether to have a lumpectomy without radiation therapy, axillary node procedure, and so on. If you have an estrogen-receptive tumor, you may also need hormonal treatment. If you have an HER-2 tumor you may be offered trastuzumab as part of your treatment plan.

There are two categories of treatment options; one is directed at the breast and regional nodes, such as lumpectomy with radiation, and the other is treatment directed at the whole body, as with systemic chemotherapy.

Full Mastectomy

In a full mastectomy the entire breast is surgically removed. A bilateral prophylactic mastectomy may be considered if you have a strong family history of breast cancer and have tested positive for the gene that predisposes you to breast cancer. Lumpectomy with radiation is a partial mastectomy with radiation therapy. Another option is a lumpectomy, radiation, and chemotherapy combination, which is recommended for breast cancers after the tumor size, grade, estrogen-receptor status, and a woman's health and age are all taken into account.

Systemic Breast Cancer Treatment / Chemotherapy

The adjuvant chemotherapy choice is one of the most difficult, because it means that chemotherapy might be recommended by your doctor but it is not imperative in your breast cancer treatment. Adjuvant chemotherapy is given as a precautionary measure, along with the primary treatment. It is a personal choice to receive it and will depend on how aggressive you want to be in your breast cancer treatment.

Alert

On the AdjuventOnline website you can put in the information about your specific breast cancer situation and the site will help guide you in your decision as to whether to have adjuvant chemotherapy (www .adjuvantonline.com).

Deciding whether to have adjuvant chemotherapy carries much responsibility, because chemotherapy has many temporary side effects some of which can be permanent life changes, such as early menopause. This may or may not be important to you, and your values can influence your decision. The challenge presented to you may find you questioning what you value in life. For example, a young woman faced with breast cancer who wants to have children may seriously have to examine the percentage of benefit of having adjuvant chemotherapy and its impact on early menopause. Another woman who has had children, or who does not wish to have children, may view this decision differently.

In general, this initial treatment decision is one of the most difficult times in the cancer experience, because there are many unknowns. Knowing that there are choices can be a stress-producing time for such an important life-sustaining decision. This is the time when gathering information about your tumor, seeking a second opinion, and seeking the advice of medical professionals in the field or family friends whose opinion you respect are extremely important to your peace of mind.

Side effects and cancer treatment will be further discussed in Chapter 5.

Fact

Never underestimate the power of your choices and what that power means to you. Your decisions about breast cancer treatment are life altering and will require determination and commitment to the choices you make. There is no right or wrong choice, but it is a personal decision, and you are in the driver's seat.

Examine Your Decision

Once you decide on your breast cancer treatment after examining all the pros and cons of your available choices, allow the whole breast cancer situation to sink in. You may want to write down the pros and cons of each of your choices and examine them on paper. Then just sit with it. Let it be present in your mind, body, and spirit and decide how it feels to you and what your inner self is telling you. Look at your decision. Does it reflect a pattern for you in how you have made other important decisions in your life? When one looks at past patterns and compares them to one's present circumstances, a similarity emerges that may help you draw on those resources you found helpful in the past.

Essential

It is said that 10 percent of life is what happens to you and 90 percent is what you decide to do with it. It is important to decide within yourself how you propose to live with your breast cancer experience.

Reflecting on your decision is important. Reflection can help you change the old patterns if you find them to be unhealthy. Or you can draw from those experiences and resources that were successful and have worked for you. Look at where you are in your life, whether you are single, married, have children, your career goals, hobbies, and what you enjoy in life. Prioritize your needs and look at your future goals for cancer treatment and beyond.

Slow Down—Make an Informed Decision

Once you are diagnosed with breast cancer, the overwhelming feeling of doing something to get rid of it permeates your mind. What to do next and the feeling that one must move quickly takes over. The reality of the progression of breast cancer and the fact that it grows slowly is often all but forgotten when you are initially diagnosed. Studies of cancer cells show that it takes about ten years for most tumors to get to a size that can be felt. Although your diagnosis seems to be an emergency, know that there is time to choose your treatment and time to go for second opinions at each stage of your breast cancer treatment. You owe it to yourself to feel comfortable with your decisions and it takes time to process the information that allows you to make those choices. For example, if the possibility of early menopause interferes with your life goals of having children, you may want to consult a specialist that has researched this area and how it relates to breast cancer prior to choosing adjuvant chemotherapy.

Usually, after breast surgery, chemotherapy and radiation will not start for four to six weeks and, although you may be tired and feeling weak from surgery, you can use this time to further investigate your options to help with your final decision-making about post-surgery treatment options.

Make the Best Decision with the Information You Have

The more knowledge you have about your tumor, the clearer your decision-making process will be. Keep in mind that human nature will have you doubting your decisions even when much time and thought has been given to them.

Alert

Remember no two breast cancer scenarios are the same. Two breast cancer tumors may be similar in size and grade and even have the same lymph node involvement, but you need to remember that your choice should be based on past experience, what is important to you, your family history, personal fears, and other unique considerations. This is why it is important not to fall into the trap of comparing your breast cancer situation with someone else's.

Some situations will challenge your choices at this vulnerable time in your life and may possibly give you some self-doubt about what you have chosen for yourself: After careful investigation, consulting doctors, family, friends, and the Internet, you have made a decision to have adjuvant chemotherapy or maybe a mastectomy with or without reconstructive surgery. Whatever the choice, the reality sets in as you live with side effects as you go through treatment, get fitted for a new bra, or deal with breast reconstruction surgery. You meet someone who had a similar experience to yours (or so it seems). She may have decided on a lumpectomy and radiation whereas you decided on a more aggressive approach including chemotherapy.

In Her Own Words

I decided to go for reconstructive surgery—did it at the same time I had my double mastectomy. Reason: I am 49 and have a long life to live. My personal appearance is very much a part of who I am. I also wanted to minimize the amount of surgeries, so going under once with two procedures was one of the best decisions I made.

—Pat, age 49, 6-month survivor

At these times, it is helpful to remember what went into your decision-making process and what the factors were at the time that convinced you to make the decisions that you did. Perhaps you wrote the pros and cons in a journal that you can refer to. Once you make your decision, don't second-guess yourself, but know you made the best decision with the information at hand.

Getting Rid of "What If?"

What if you had different biological parents? What if you lived your life differently? You think to yourself that maybe if you didn't drink so much diet soda, or drink alcohol, or eat high fat foods, you wouldn't be dealing with your breast cancer diagnosis right now. What if you had the perfect life and lived in a stress-free world and the environment was clean and eco-friendly, would things be different?

All of this is a waste of your precious energy. It is an exercise in futility to dwell on the whys and what ifs. It is more productive to get on with the here-and-now and by doing so you will be better equipped to face the challenges that lie ahead, both physically and emotionally.

⌶ Essential

You have so much to deal with in the day-to-day occurrences that come with breast cancer treatment that looking at all the other possible scenarios will only overwhelm you. Taking one day at a time will help you keep on track and focused on the situation at hand.

Try Not to Jump Ahead of Where You Are

When going through breast cancer treatment, many thoughts, fears, and concerns race through your head. Why you? Are you doing the right thing? What if there is a better way to go with your treatment choice? What if it doesn't work? What about the children? What will happen to them? How will you get through it? It's as though all your thoughts are in a dryer, spinning around and around out of control, and then stopping from time to time. When you stop to think, the dryer opens and everything seems to come out at once. This is when you feel overwhelmed. If this sounds familiar to you, you are not alone. One way to deal with it is to look at your current situation in pieces. Deal only with what is confronting you now. It may be getting through your first day of chemotherapy and how your body will react to it, or the first day you wear a headscarf or wig out in public.

CHAPTER 5

Treatment Options and Side Effects

Fear of the unknown is what is often the most troubling. Not knowing what to expect can make the experience of cancer treatment more uncertain and promote anxiety. One way to counteract that uncertainty is to learn about the various options of cancer treatment available to you and their side effects. The three primary breast cancer treatments are surgery (whether a lumpectomy/ partial mastectomy, full radical mastectomy), medical therapy (such as chemotherapy and hormonal therapy), and radiation. The sequencing of the surgery, chemotherapy, and radiation, varies depending on your specific situation. Your doctor will explain the recommended treatment plan to you. The goal of this chapter is to provide you with an overview of breast cancer treatment, its side effects, and some helpful hints to live within those side effects as comfortably as possible.

Surgery

The goal of surgery is to remove the tumor. Breast cancer surgery varies from a partial to a total mastectomy, (or breast-conserving surgery, such as a lumpectomy.) Which one is done depends on what your breasts mean to you, your body image, the size of the tumor, the type, stage, and characteristics of the tumor viewed at the cellular level, and tumor tissue from your breast biopsy report.

For example, if you had a type of breast cancer most apt to recur in the other breast or the probability is high for recurrence, you have a strong family history, and genetic testing comes back positive for the gene, you may opt for prophylactic bilateral mastectomies. Remember, most women will do well with a lumpectomy. Getting a bilateral mastectomy is actually fairly rare. Again, this is a personal decision that requires investigation.

A lumpectomy is usually done as day surgery at a surgical center or the hospital unless complications arise during the surgery. For a partial mastectomy, an overnight hospital stay is likely; a full mastectomy usually involves a hospital stay of one to two days, and a mastectomy with reconstructive surgery will generally require even longer hospitalization. Note that you need to let your surgeon and oncologist know if there is no support system at home or if there are any special considerations that may hinder your recovery. Perhaps you are the primary caretaker for a disabled child or other family member. This may alter your hospital stay requirements and you may need to stay an extra day. However, you may need to look at your insurance coverage and discuss it with your doctor. We will discuss insurance coverage in Chapter 6, including how to work with your coverage.

Surgery is stress-producing and a violation to your system. Breast cancer surgery has added stresses and, unlike most other surgeries, has more of an emotional impact associated with it. For example, when you have stomach or heart surgery, you can focus on the healing of your incision and perhaps consider some lifestyle changes in your recovery process. With breast cancer, surgery is often only the beginning of your treatment plan. It seems as though you need to not only heal from your surgery, but also think about what lies ahead in your treatment, and deal with a life-threatening illness and the physical and psychological factors associated with it.

Prepare yourself for your surgery by keeping your mind, body, and spirit focused and healthy. Prior to surgery, you can expect to meet with an anesthesiologist and it is your responsibility to share any pertinent medical history, previous experience with anesthesia or the experiences of your immediate family regarding anesthesia. The anesthesiologist will be looking for clues as to what type of anesthesia to use and your medication reaction history is important to determining this.

Post-surgery is the first time you will have a clear snapshot of your breast cancer situation and it is a more critical time for you, along with your doctor, to determine further treatment choices.

Side Effects

Post-surgery, expect to have discomfort in your breast and under your arm if an axillary dissection was done. Many breast cancer centers offer a pillow to use under your arm to alleviate this discomfort.

 In Her Own Words

When the lumpectomy did not get all the margins and the tumor was larger than they thought, I had the choice of another lumpectomy or a mastectomy. I had DCIS [ductal carcinoma in situ] in one breast and it was not invasive. I met with a medical oncologist, a radiation oncologist, and a plastic surgeon about my choices. I got all the facts of reoccurrence. I decided to get a double mastectomy with reconstruction at age 42. For me it was what I needed to do to have the best chance of never having to deal with this again.

—Theresa, age 46, 4-year survivor

After having surgery, you may notice a numbness or tingling sensation in the affected breast. This occurs because nerves were damaged during the surgery. No further breast cancer treatment can begin until the surgical area heals and there are no signs of infection. You can expect a four- to six-week wait, but this also depends on your healing ability and your readiness to begin treatment.

Other possible side effects that may result from your surgery include infection at the site of surgery or more serious infections that spread through the body via the blood system.

Reconstructive Surgery

A total or simple mastectomy operation involves the removal of the entire breast but does not cut away any lymph nodes or muscle tissue. The surgeon tunnels under the skin all the way up to the collarbone to remove the breast. Drains are placed in the incision to prevent fluid building up in the empty space. If you are not having immediate reconstruction surgery, then the incision is closed and you will have a bulky wraparound dressing. The breast's nerve supply has been cut so the area around the scar will be numb permanently. Later a volunteer from the American Cancer Society's Reach for Recovery program will visit either in the hospital or at your home to discuss prosthesis and other fears or concerns. The Reach to Recovery volunteer has experienced breast cancer surgery and understands from a personal perspective about your experience. Resources and helpful tips are shared at this visit and, most importantly, it gives you the opportunity to share your concerns and fears and about the physical changes that are occurring.

If you opt for reconstructive surgery over the use of prosthetics (and this option is available to you) reconstructive surgery can be done in various ways. The breast can be surgically reconstructed using artificial substances such as silicone or your own body tissue.

The silicone implant (the simplest reconstructive method) is placed behind the pectoral muscle and then the skin is sewn over it, almost like a pocket. Then, where an implant has been placed under the skin, saline is injected slowly over a period of six months until you reach the size you want. Then the expander implant is removed and replaced with the silicone sack.

In a procedure using your own tissues, called a myocutaneous flap, a flap of skin, muscle, and fat is taken from your back or your abdomen to reconstruct the breast. In this type of surgery, tissue is taken with a feeding artery and vein and then planted in the breast and sewn over with the blood supply still intact. This feels more like your own breast because it is your own tissue that is being used, but it will still not have the sensation of a normal breast. For this type of surgery you can expect to stay in the hospital for four to five days.

When you meet with your plastic surgeon to discuss breast reconstruction, it is a good idea to bring someone with you to your appointment. It is difficult to comprehend all that is being said and having another set of ears can be helpful when taking notes and deciding on the reconstructive surgery that is best for you. It is also a good idea to ask the plastic surgeon to show you before and after pictures of her work, to give you a good idea of what to expect. Also the plastic surgeon will explain that initially you will not have a nipple but that can be created at a later time by various methods such as tattooing or taking skin from your thigh, which darkens when it is transplanted.

The decision to have reconstructive surgery is a personal choice, and there are many factors to consider when making the decision as to which type of surgery you will have. Psychologically, it may be easier to accept losing your breasts when you have it done at the same time as your mastectomy and you see that there is a replacement there. On the other hand, it may delay the adjustment process to the reality that you have had breast cancer. Many breast experts favor immediate reconstruction. For many women, the ease of not wearing a prosthesis and looking normal in a bathing suit and in their clothes offsets the time and effort it takes to go through reconstructive surgery. The choice of having reconstructive surgery at a later date is also a viable option if a woman is not ready emotionally or physically at the time of her breast surgery.

Chemotherapy

Chemotherapy is a systemic approach to breast cancer treatment, in which chemicals are introduced into your bloodstream with the intention of killing cancer cells. But chemotherapy is not selective in which cells are affected, so healthy noncancerous cells may be damaged as well. Chemotherapy affects other fast-growing cells in the body. This contributes to the hair loss that is one of the most feared and thought about side effects of chemotherapy. More importantly, chemotherapy also affects the rapidly dividing cells of the bone marrow, which is where your red blood cells, white blood cells, and platelets are manufactured on an ongoing basis. These make up the life force of your blood and influence your health in many ways.

In Her Own Words

Before chemo treatments begin, you'll be given a prescription for anti-anxiety meds, the filling of which is optional. In my opinion, it should be mandatory. Granted it is different for everyone, but in my experience taking these drugs was extremely helpful until two months after treatment.

—Mary, age 51, 4-year survivor

Red blood cells are the oxygen-carrying cells that circulate in your body's system and keep it working. A low red-cell count contributes to feelings of low energy and weakness. A low white blood cell count affects your body's ability to fight infection. Conversely, if the white blood cell counts are high, it shows that the body is fighting some type of foreign body, such as an infection. Because chemotherapy affects normal cell division, it is given in cycles, so that the blood-producing cells in the bone marrow can recover (and you can begin to recover as well) before the next cycle of treatment.

Routinely, prior to receiving chemotherapy, blood work is done in the doctor's office to monitor your cell counts, to make sure you are well enough to receive your next infusion or injection. During your course of chemotherapy, your treatment may be delayed because your blood counts have not been given enough time to recover.

Alert

It may come as a surprise to you that if your chemotherapy is delayed because of your blood counts, you may be disappointed rather than relieved. This is because you want things to go as scheduled. Remember that the immune system varies from individual to individual and the goal is to kill cancer cells, but not at the expense of your immune system being so depleted that the bone marrow isn't able to recover.

Chemotherapy Drugs

The concept behind chemotherapy is to interfere with cancer cell growth at various stages of its growth. The term *chemotherapy* refers to the infusion of drugs that can kill cells, hopefully more cancer than normal cells. Chemotherapy drugs are classified based on how they work. Some of the main types of cytotoxic (cell-killing) chemotherapy are:

- *Alkylating drugs* kill cancer cells by directly attacking DNA, the genetic makeup of the genes. (Example: cyclophosphamide, brand-name Cytokan)
- *Antimetabolites* interfere with production of DNA and keep the cells from growing and multiplying. (Example: 5-fluorouracil; also referred to as 5-FU)
- *Antitumor antibiotics* which are made from natural substances, interfere with cell functions, production of DNA, and cell proteins. (Examples: doxorubicin and bleomycin)
- *Plant alkaloids* prevent cells from dividing normally. (Examples: vinblastine and vincristine)

This list gives an indication of why combination chemotherapy recipes are used—each drug affects the cancer cells differently. One may interfere with the DNA in the cell and cell division while another drug may act on how fast cells divide. Another way to think of chemotherapy is to refer to treatment with drugs as the "medical" therapy of breast cancer. There are now multiple categories of medicines used, including cytotoxic chemotherapy, hormonal approaches, and antibodies such as trastuzumab and bevacizumab. There will be more categories of medicines as understanding of cell biology increases.

What to Expect at Your Treatments

Once the combination recipe has been decided on, you will be scheduled for your chemotherapy treatments. Chemotherapy is administered by infusion or injection, and usually requires a course of treatments over a period of weeks. Infusion treatment can take a long time, and you might need to prepare to spend the better part of or an entire day at the clinic (see Appendix D for a list of what to bring to your chemotherapy appointments).

The Decision to Have Chemotherapy

Early stage breast cancer offers many options for treatment and treatment recommendations are based on lymph node involvement, the size of the tumor, the grade of the tumor, and other cell characteristics seen under the microscope that suggest the behavior of the cancer (for instance, it is likely to have already spread to other parts of the body). However, you are an equal partner in the decision to have chemotherapy and you need to carefully review your options with your doctor, along with your support system or family, and then make your own decision after these detailed discussions.

Age, life goals, medical history, family history, philosophy, and personal needs are all important considerations that may weigh into the decision on whether to have adjuvant chemotherapy. When there is no lymph node involvement, some chemotherapy choices considered are four cycles of AC, which is short for the combination of doxorubicin (Adriamycin) and cyclophosphamide

(Cytoxan); or six cycles of CMF, which is short for the combination of cyclophosphamide (Cytoxan), methotrexate, and 5-fluorourcal (5-FU). These chemotherapy regimes occur about every three weeks. However, chemotherapy regimens are changing all the time. Coauthor Dr. Stewart favors an approach that encourages participation in national clinical trials or use of a "standard" regimen that has been validated in national clinical trials.

 ## In Her Own Words

Adequate hydration is the key to managing chemotherapy. Drink as much water as you can, start the day before chemo and continue for three days after your treatment. Staying hydrated prevents many side effects and helps circulate the medications to every area of the body. Antiemetics are medications to prevent nausea and vomiting; they are extremely effective. Take these medications with the first signs of nausea.

—Suzanne, age 52, one-year survivor

Chemotherapy is an option with node-positive breast cancer, especially if the tumor is estrogen-receptor negative. The chemotherapy is given in addition to other treatment, such as radiation, and hormone therapy, depending on the situation. Also, an individual's age or medical status may prohibit chemotherapy treatment. An oncologist may recommend surgery first for a case of advanced local breast cancer disease. And in metastatic breast cancer that has spread to other organs, whether the tumor is estrogen-receptor positive or negative may determine the treatment regimen recommended.

Whatever treatment you choose, once the decision is made, keep your goals in mind.

Side Effects

Side effects of chemotherapy can include hair loss, yellowing of the skin, brittle nails, susceptibility to infection, nausea and vomiting, headaches, depression, loss of appetite, mouth sores, and fatigue. (This is not a complete list. Consult your doctor if you experience other serious side effects of your chemotherapy.) You may experience some or all of these side effects, but fortunately most of these are temporary. The most common are mouth sores, fatigue, and vomiting. Mouth sores can be treated with a non-alcohol mouthwash to avoid irritation of the lining of the mouth, but fatigue might be the result of anemia, and may indicate that you'll need medication to get more iron into your blood. You might find that stomach upset and vomiting can exacerbate the dehydration also typically experienced by chemotherapy patients, and so you'll need to request anti-nausea medication from your doctor. Other homeopathic approaches will be discussed in Chapter 11.

What Are Clinical Trials and Are They for Me?

Research studies known as clinical trials test new drugs and treatments and compare them to current treatments. In the United States, patients have great access to treatment trials, which are organized treatment plans that collect data regarding effectiveness and side effects. If you are considering participating in a clinical trial for your cancer treatment, there is information available to you from your doctor's office and someone will be assigned to explain the trial in depth. This is again a personal choice. You may not see any benefit from it. But the findings may result in better breast cancer treatment in the future for someone else. Treatment in the context of a clinical trial should generally be considered a good opportunity.

The primary questions researchers want to answer are:

- Does this treatment work?
- Does it work better than the treatment we are using now?
- What side effects does it cause?
- Do the benefits outweigh the risks?
- Which patients are most likely to benefit from this treatment?

You may want to be included in a clinical trial, and discussing this as an option may help you get a better understanding of breast cancer treatment. You are not obliged to take part in the clinical trial after you have inquired about it, so it can't hurt to ask.

Hormone Therapies

Hormone therapy uses drugs to inhibit the activity of hormones such as estrogen and progesterone, that support the growth and spread of cancer cells. Hormonal systemic treatment of breast cancer involves taking a pill by mouth, usually twice a day. For estrogen-receptor negative tumors, or tumors not fed by estrogen, one would not consider hormone therapy. Tamoxifen is the most common hormone treatment used and has been available for use the longest. It is a selective estrogen receptor modulator, which means it has anti-estrogen effects on hormone-receptor positive breast cancer and estrogenic effects on some other tissues, such as bones and the uterus.

Another class of hormonal agents, aromatase inhibitors, includes anastrozole (Arimidex), letrozole (Femara) and exemestane (Aromasin). In post-menopausal women, fatty tissue can be converted into estrogen by the using an enzyme called aromatase, and aromatase inhibitors block this process. In addition to aromatase inhibitors, there is an approach to destroying estrogen receptors called fulvestrant (Faslodex), which is given by monthly injections.

Side Effects

Serious side effects of various hormone therapies include increased risks for other cancers, bone thinning and osteoporosis, and abnormal clotting of the blood. Side effects with hormone therapy can include weight gain, hot flashes, vaginal dryness, and nausea.

Radiation Therapy

Radiation therapy uses high-intensity X-rays to kill unstable cancer cells, while leaving normal cells to regenerate themselves during and after treatment. With breast cancer, radiation is usually a treatment of choice along with surgery unless a radical or full mastectomy has been done. Whatever the recommendations, make sure you understand it and it feels right to you. Radiation treatment is an exact science, the body's response to it and individual cancer cells' response varies.

Your nutritional status is important during this time because the radiation treatment requires much energy on the cellular level. You may come out of treatment feeling like you have spent a long day at the beach, but radiation treatment is certainly not a day at the beach. Your body will need proper nourishment to replenish your energy during radiation treatment. (Diet is discussed in Chapter 9).

What to Expect at Your Appointments

The radiation oncologist will be doing a treatment plan for your radiation. He will first see you on a consultation visit, where a medical history and physical are done, and all your reports, such as pathology report, mammogram, MRI, and co-existing illnesses, will be reviewed. The radiation oncologist uses cell grade, type, and stage of breast cancer as well as size and the body area to be radiated to determine how much radiation should be given and where. He then determines the dose levels and how long the treatments should be. To do these he follows guidelines used by radiologists from clinical trials.

Your first appointment is the longest and usually lasts one to two hours. Precise mapping of your breast will be done through a simulator with a laser localization system. This is linked with a CAT scan of your body surface so that the right amount of radiation is delivered to the correct areas. The actual planning occurs after your visit. The radiation oncologist and a simulator therapist will mark both the simulator and the CAT scan of your body to link them. Data is electronically transferred to a medical physics department, where physicists and technicians create the treatment plan based on the radiology oncologist's prescription of dose and number of treatments. The goal is to develop a plan with radiation beams and angles that will allow for the best possible coverage of the affected breast and lymph node area. There are other specialized techniques to promote even distribution to all tissues when needed. The treatment plan is then sent back to the radiology oncologist to review and approve and then the completed plan is electronically sent to the radiation machine.

 Alert

Mapping is done by a simulator and involves a technician along with the radiology oncologist to draw lines on your breast to indicate where the radiation is aimed. These lines are put on with semi-permanent markers, but during the summer months sweating can diminish the markings. Don't worry, it is all calculated and the radiology oncologist or the technician will be able to re-draw them. Also, the hand-drawn lines are not really the marks the treatment machine uses, rather the tattoos are used to line things up.

Some doctors will also use permanent tattoos to designate the area for radiation treatment. These dots are very tiny but to the one with breast cancer they may have an emotional impact—a permanent reminder that you have had radiation treatment. The radiation treatment usually goes on for six and a half weeks. A boosting dose may be used when the tumor margins are close, so additional radiation to that area is done as a safety precaution, the goal of radiation treatment being to eliminate any microscopic cancer cells that may have been left behind.

The second visit, which typically occurs four to five days after the consultation visit, is the verification visit. A test is made to make sure what was calculated in the physicists' department is what you are getting on the machine. The radiology oncologist digitally reconstructs the breast by giving a small dose, which looks similar to an x-ray, and makes final recommendations based on these findings.

The third visit is when your radiation treatments typically begin. The process may vary among breast radiation centers, but the basic guidelines are the same. The radiation process is painless, and occurs at the same time each day, usually Monday through Friday. The entire time of direct radiation is usually less than one minute. The technician will come in and position you, then leave the room and give the radiation. This will happen again or until the desired amount of radiation is given. Often, getting to the local hospital or radiation oncology department on a daily basis interferes with your work schedule or lifestyle and is more of an annoyance than the actual treatments. During radiation treatment, it is important to remain still, so it may help to use an iPod or MP3 player to listen to music while you are receiving radiation.

The Radiation Treatment

It is a good idea to bring someone for support the first time you have radiation treatment, since you don't know what to expect and it can be emotionally draining. When you have radiation treatments, you will change into a hospital johnny from the waist up. You can't wear jewelry around your neck. This includes body piercing jewelry on your breast; you may want to check with your radiology oncologist about head and neck piercings. For changing purposes, it is easier for you to wear an outfit that is two pieces. You will lie on a radiation table with a radiation machine above you. A plastic or Styrofoam pillow is placed under your head. The radiation is given at different angles. The technician will position you, leave the room, and turn on the radiation machine. You can talk with the technician through an intercom system if necessary or if you feel anxious. If you are being treated for metastatic cancer, then treatments are different and the goal is for pain relief or symptom relief. A smaller dose is usually given in ten to fifteen treatments over two-and-a-half weeks.

 Fact

Skin care is important during the time you are undergoing radiation treatment. It is recommended that you use mild soap and no deodorant. You can use a small amount of cornstarch if needed, or go to a natural food store and ask for a non-aluminum deodorant. Be very careful when reading the label. Another natural skin product that is allowed during radiation treatments is aloe vera lotion. Again read the label for all ingredients.

One side effect that may occur in some women is a condition called costochondritis, which is an inflammation in the chest where the ribs and breastbone (sternum) connect. Usually this can be treated with Tylenol, aspirin, or another anti-inflammatory medication.

Fatigue is a common side effect of radiation and varies from individual to individual. It is important to remain physically active during your radiation treatments, within moderation, so that you can continue after your treatments are completed. This will help you to heal and improve your general feeling of well-being.

Partial Breast Radiation

Partial breast radiation is given to a smaller portion of the breast. There are several ways to deliver partial breast radiation. For example, temporarily implanting radioactive seeds into the breast area (either with a balloon technique or using multiple implanted tubes called interstitial brachytherapy) and external beam treatments. This is currently being studied in a national clinical trial. One approach being tested is accelerated partial breast radiation, in which only the area of the tumor, not the whole breast, is treated in fewer days than the usual five to six weeks.

Which Treatment Option Is Best for You?

The team approach is often the best way to decide on your treatment plan. It is important to recognize that the decision ultimately lies with you and that to make the best decision takes time and energy. Solicit input from your doctor and your support system, and balance this with your personal values, wants, and needs, and the reality of having breast cancer. As mentioned earlier, the size, grade, lymph node involvement, stage of breast cancer, and estrogen-receptor status factor into your recommended breast cancer treatment plan. Depending on how aggressive you want to be with your cancer treatment, you can further investigate other bio-markers and tests that may give you the additional information needed for you to choose your treatment. Depending on the importance you place on your breast, consider whether to have a breast-conserving lumpectomy or mastectomy, and then what type of mastectomy (modified or radical). Such decisions will vary with each individual.

Making the Right Decision for You

Breaking down your larger decisions into steps or parts can be helpful, as can attempting to view your breast cancer situation with a detached perspective. In order to determine a smart and prudent course of action, you have to learn all you can about your breast cancer diagnosis and tumor. Be an expert on your tumor's size, stage, lymph node status, estrogen-receptor status, and HER-2 status, and be knowledgeable on all the treatments available to you as well as possible clinical trials, if you are interested.

Alternatively, listen to what your body is telling you. It is important to realize that for the body to form cancer cells and a tumor, something within the body has changed. Be sensitive to physiological changes that are occurring. You may feel fine now physically, but you may want to choose a course of action that is proactive as opposed to reactive.

Only after you have explored your treatment options; sought the advice of medical professionals, family, and friends; and have looked to the spiritual resources that have helped you in the past will you know your choices are the right ones.

It is only the combination of mind, body, and spirit that makes a decision feel whole and complete. Afford yourself the time to examine each decision in solitude and have peace of mind about your decision before you go forward.

CHAPTER 6

Personal Resources and Support Systems

You ask yourself, "How am I going to get through this?" This may be the first time in your life that you've had to take a survey of your resources and your assets, both personally and financially. The time has come to look at your net worth in personal resources, such as family and friends, as well as the financial and work resources that may help you get through your breast cancer treatments. Included in the asset management are your healthcare providers, who become part of your extended circle of support during this time. Exploring your own sense of spirituality and what it means to you will be the least tangible aspect of your survey, but one that can give you the most support and provide meaning to your experience.

Know Your Support Systems

Emily Dickinson said, "My friends are my estate." Ralph Waldo Emerson said, "A friend may well be reckoned the masterpiece of nature." Each of you living with breast cancer will discover the power of friends. You will witness the love, companionship, and the caring impact of friends. There are some universal truths to friendship and support. One is that friends can truly make a difference in your life, especially in times of need. It is one way to know who your friends truly are.

Friends have different roles. Some friends will be ahead of you, anticipating your every need, some will be behind you, picking up the pieces, and some will walk beside you in silence. At the end of your breast cancer journey, your real friends will be there and a bond will remain forever. You will also meet new friends—perhaps someone who is going through the breast cancer experience at the same time or someone you have talked to who has lived through the breast cancer experience and has been a support to you.

Essential

"You will have many friends around you and it is similar to running a race. Everyone runs their race in various ways: some run real fast in the beginning because that's their pace, some run slow and steady, and some run slow in the beginning and catch up when others are tired and weak. Your real friends will be there at the end no matter what pace you set. You will lose some along the way and gain some along the way, but the end result is the same. Your true friends will be there alongside you whatever the pace."

—An Anonymous Friend

Friends tend to be more objective than family by virtue of their relationship to you. Family members, in many ways, have no choice other than to be there. You have a place in your family that has already been set. You may be the one who holds things together, the peacemaker, and the "make-nice" person in the family unit. You may be the caretaker for everyone—your children, friends, coworkers, and extended family. The amazing thing about breast cancer is that it doesn't change who you are, but it may change the circumstances and roles that you play in the family. If you have been the nurturer in the family, then being the receiver of help may be a very difficult role for you. And vice versa—if you are the one who is the strength in the family, it will be difficult to be in a position in which family members now have to give you strength.

The systems theory can be easily applied to family life and what your role is in the family. One of the main tenets of systems theory is that the whole is greater than the sum of the parts. When one family member has a life-threatening illness such as breast cancer, then other parts or members will be disrupted and the system will need to adapt and change to make the family system work for you.

In Her Own Words

To allow for beautifully colored hair, we allow for processing time. After the initial shock of a cancer diagnosis, processing time is essential. Give yourself the time, space, and freedom to experience the full gamut of emotions. Afterward you will be ready to embrace the highlights of your beautiful new life.

—Michelle, age 38, 1-year survivor

Take an inventory of your support system, whether it is made up of family, or family and friends, or only friends. Remember, as Emily Dickinson said, they will be your "estate," or your assets, during your breast cancer treatments.

Bring Someone You Respect to Your Appointments

A good rule of thumb is to bring someone you trust and respect to your appointments because when your doctor is talking about your breast cancer and treatment it is hard to take in all the information. This time, it is not about someone you know, but it is about you. You do not have to choose someone from your family or someone with a medical background to come with you to your appointments. The person you choose can be anyone you feel comfortable with. He or she simply needs to be an extra set of ears so that you can discuss with them your breast cancer and so better understand its treatment and your goals after your appointment.

This is one time in your life that you need to put yourself first. You can pick and choose who you want with you when you go to your appointments, chemotherapy treatments, or radiation treatments. Some of you may choose to go alone because that is what makes you the most comfortable. Whatever helps you get through treatments is the way to go. You may want to make the most of your wealth of friends and have different friends help with different things. You may learn on your journey that the least suspected family member or friend was the person that helped you the most. This is a time in your life that you come first.

Friends and Family Will Keep You Going in the Midst of Adversity

Let your friends and family help you. This is the all-important message that will help carry you through your breast cancer treatment. Assemble your team of support and say yes to offers of help. The offers may be as simple as making you a home-cooked meal, taking a walk in the park with you, taking your children for a short time, or even taking them for a sleepover to give you a break from your everyday responsibilities.

 In Her Own Words

Finding a support system was very easy for me. I didn't have to find it, it found me. My friends and family were incredible. Another person that walked into my life was a wonderful woman, Christine, who started a wellness group with the local hospital's breast center. I was in the first group. We called ourselves the "A Team." I would encourage anyone to look into this program.

—Debra, age 47, 4-year survivor

Practice saying yes to others' offers of help. Many women going through breast cancer treatment have shared incredible stories about the caring people in their lives who have helped them. Give someone who cares about you that opportunity and gift to be of service to you. The friends and family around you often feel helpless and want to be in some small way a support to you. On the other hand, not all friends and family are in a position to give and be of support. That's okay too. Enjoy the willing and the able, because they will be your greatest gift while you are going through breast cancer treatment and recovery.

Health Care Providers as Partners

Your new world will seem to be made up of so many appointments, cancer treatments, and follow-up appointments that it will be hard to keep track. The medical world that may have been so foreign to you except for your regular yearly checkups is now consuming your life. You are very busy with coordinating your medical care, participating in medical decisions, and just going to appointments. It is hard to believe that you can fit in the day-to-day responsibilities of your work and family life.

When receiving cancer treatment, whether it is chemotherapy, radiation, or hormone therapy, you will be in contact with many doctors, nurses, and health care professionals. If there is a major breast cancer center in your area, you may want to visit and tap into its resources. For example, breast centers usually have social workers who can help you deal with some of the emotional issues that arise from breast cancer treatment. The hospital where you are receiving treatment will have personnel who will help with insurance coverage issues and in-house social workers or case managers who will be available to you. Often you have to be proactive and ask the question for the support to be activated.

These health care professionals, whether they are dietitians, nurses, physical therapists, or doctors, are there to be your partners during your breast cancer treatment and recovery. You need to think of them in a way that promotes communication and relationship-building so that the partnership will work. Again, the partnership is as good as all the partners and their ability to work together. Remember that you are the only consistent partner and at the center of the health care team—the true expert on what your needs will be.

In Her Own Words

What truly helped me through all of this was my faith. I went back to church when I was diagnosed and I realized with the help of my priest that we do not have "map quest" for our lives, something bigger than us has the plan. We need to turn our will over to God. We have no control over some things in life, only how we deal with them.

—Theresa, age 46, 4-year survivor

Spiritual Strength: Build Upon Your Spiritual Self

Many medical professionals, psychologists, philosophers, and religious people recognize the power of faith. Your spiritual beliefs make a difference in how you view your breast cancer experience and you may believe that even this experience is part of a larger plan. Whatever your beliefs are, building on your spiritual self can be a source of great strength and support. Belief in a higher being can give you hope in the deepest, most difficult times in your life. Often faith grows stronger in times of need. Scientists have discovered that a feeling of hopefulness promotes healing and that faith often releases endorphins in the body. These endorphins are similar to those that circulate in runners and give them a "high" after running. These circulating endorphins have healing and pain-relief power. Building upon your spiritual self can include praying, meditating, relaxation practices, and being one with a higher being. The specifics of how you view faith and what your faith is are not the important pieces of spirituality. Spirituality is seeing inner beauty in yourself, others, and the world around you. It is seeing without seeing. It is a felt sense of purpose in life.

The holistic approach to breast cancer recognizes that the human experience is made up of body, mind, and spirit, and they all work together so that a person may find peace within herself, her relationship to others, and her place in the world. Though the mind-body connection has been clearly proven to create health or illness, the spiritual aspect of health continues to be the hardest to explain. It is not tangible, but it can be as personally powerful as any medical breakthrough or treatment in breast cancer. While being a spiritual person or using holistic approaches may not physically affect your cancer, it can certainly help you feel better, cope better, and get more out of life.

Essential

It is important to realize that you do not have to be involved in an organized religion to develop your spirituality. It can be what you want it to be. However, many people have a support community associated with their religious faith that is a source of strength for them. The choice is yours in how you decide to maintain or rediscover your spiritual self.

Financial Resources

Few things have as big an impact on your financial hopes and dreams for a good life as having a life-threatening illness like breast cancer. You may have heard one of your elder relatives say that if you don't have health, you have nothing. This statement never feels as true as when you are actively going through breast cancer treatment. The future is unknown, your prognosis is sketchy, and nothing you ever did in the past, like saving, or dreaming of retirement, makes sense to you right now. That job you may have been dissatisfied with looks good when you think you may not ever go back to it and your normal way of life. Your job is part of your everyday life and now that you need cancer treatment, your work seems to revolve around doctor's appointments. This seems to be the new job that you did not want to have.

This is when your financial assets and liabilities become part of your breast cancer experience. Once again, you have that overwhelming feeling and many questions bombard you: Will you be able to work? Can you make ends meet? What will your health insurance pay and what will you be responsible for? If you do not have health insurance, will you be able to get the necessary care?

Health Insurance

If you have health insurance, the first thing you need to do is call the customer service number that is usually on the back of your insurance card and find out what your insurance covers. You particularly want to know if you need to use preferred providers to get the full coverage. For example, if your insurance is a health maintenance organization (HMO) or a preferred provider organization (PPO), there may be certain rules that apply to get the most out of your health care benefits. Some insurers pay at a 100 percent rate when you use their preferred providers and give you the option of going out of their network at a reduced rate of coverage. A customer service representative at your insurance provider can help you figure out which doctors are in your network.

Health care has evolved into a tightly controlled managed care process in which the insurer may manage your cancer treatment by reviewing hospital-stay days and high-cost drug treatments. Coverage varies for medical treatment and where the place of coverage will be. If you are in a hospital setting, there are case managers who will assist you in finding out what your insurance coverage is and what to expect for coverage. A case manager is often an advo-cate for you, who works with the health care team and the insur-ance company to meet your needs. Too often, you may find your health insurance does not cover all your expenses and you may find yourself incurring expenses that you did not expect.

 Fact

> Determine what type of health insurance you have: Is it an indemnity plan or a managed health care product? Indemnity health plans allow you to go anywhere for your breast cancer treatments and have fewer restrictions, but they are also expensive and not very common in the current health care environment.

Breast cancer treatment has a high cost associated with it, including chemotherapy, drugs, radiation treatments, prosthesis, and reconstructive surgery. You may find yourself paying out of pocket for some of your treatment. It is not uncommon to reach the maximum deductible of your insurance coverage, so it is wise for you to find out up-front what that will be. Many hospitals and breast cancer centers have financial support people that you can speak with about insurance coverage and what you will be respon-sible for financially.

Essential

> Most health insurers now are managed-care products that require you to comply with their rules for optimizing your coverage. Most insur-ance companies require prior approval before any surgery or proce-dures and many have a co-pay, which is the amount that the individual is responsible for. Remember that all policies have an out-of-pocket maximum and once that deductible is met you will not have to pay out of pocket.

All insurance companies have customer relations personnel who can help you with your individual policy coverage and are available to answer questions about your coverage. Case managers are available through your insurer and can assist you in choosing preferred providers in your HMO or PPO network to get full coverage. They can also tell you how to make choices that comply with their requirements of notification and prior approval, so as not to jeopardize your benefits. Once you have breast cancer, it can be difficult to get health insurance on your own, depending on which state you live in. Health insurance through your employer can be extended under COBRA laws for eighteen months after you are not working, but even then the premiums are often steep for individuals who are not working but are incurring high medical costs.

If You Don't Have Health Insurance

If you have no health insurance, you may want to speak with your doctor or the hospital where you are being treated. Depending on your financial status, you may be eligible for state- or government-funded health insurance. Most major hospitals also have free-care applications that you may be eligible for. You can ask to speak with a social worker or financial representative at the hospital to make arrangements for payment. Many cancer patients who need financial support are eligible for government programs such as Medicare and Medicaid. To be eligible for Medicare benefits, you need to be disabled from work for three years. Medicaid is also available, but has many restrictions associated with it and often breast cancer patients who are younger and still able to work find themselves not meeting Medicaid's strict financial criteria, but still struggling to make ends meet. If you find yourself in this situation, ask to speak to a social worker at the breast cancer center where you are receiving services. She can give you advice and help you apply for financial aid for your health care coverage or help you to find out if there are any grants available to help you.

Fact

Social Security pays benefits to people who cannot work because they have a medical condition that is expected to last at least one year or result in death. To apply for Social Security disability benefits go to *www.socialsecurity.gov* or call 1-800-772-1213. There are disability starter kits available online if you feel that you may be eligible for disability benefits at *www.socialsecurity.gov/disability*.

Medicaid is a health insurance program financed and run jointly by the federal and state governments for low-income people who do not have the money to pay for health care. Each state has its own guidelines and it is state administered. To find out if you are eligible for Medicaid, go to the Medicaid office in your state to learn about income eligibility and coverage.

Employment Benefits/Resources

What is available when you tap into your employee benefits varies from employer to employer. One consistent piece is the Family Medical Leave Act (FMLA) of 1993, which under federal law provides employees with up to twelve weeks of unpaid leave for their own serious illness, the birth or adoption of a child, or care of a seriously ill child, spouse, or parent. Depending on your company's policy, the definition of eligible employees may vary for length of employment and part time status. For purposes of the FMLA, a "serious health condition" is any illness, injury, impairment, or physical or mental condition involving inpatient care or continuing treatment by a health-care provider. Some states have their own FMLA, which may provide different and better benefits than the federal law, so check your state law.

Breast cancer treatment is covered under the FMLA, but it is up to the individual whether to take a full leave or part-time leave to accommodate breast cancer treatments. And that decision must be approved by a doctor. Many women receive much support in their work environment and working provides a distraction during treatments, as well as keeping a sense of normalcy in their lives. Once again, knowing yourself and what will be of help to you needs to be at the core of how you want to proceed. You can always change your decision if it is not working for you. You may find that keeping up with the normal work day is too stressful while going through cancer treatments or you may be experiencing many side effects from treatment that make you feel as though you are not pulling your weight at work.

Generally, FMLA leave is unpaid; however, you can usually use your accrued sick time and vacation time first. During your leave, your employer will continue to pay into your health benefits so you will be responsible for paying your portion. It is very important to keep up with payments so that your insurance benefits do not lapse. Breast cancer treatment is very costly and you must keep on top of it. If you are unable to do this, assign someone you trust to take care of this for you.

The first thing to do when you are ready is go to your human resources department at work to find out what your benefits are. You may have short-term disability or long-term disability that you may want to access. If you are going to request a leave, make sure you understand the stipulations of the FMLA. Most employers will require documentation of your request and medical certification from your physician periodically and will also need to be notified of any changes of your status or extensions. You must inform your employer of your status and when you intend to return to work. Your employer will want to hear from you periodically and will work with you on your return. Initially your doctor will need to clear you medically to return to work and you may only be able to work part time. This will also have to be worked out with your human resources department and your supervisor. The decision to work and how much, whether full time or part time, during and after breast cancer treatment varies from individual to individual depending on her circumstances.

At the end of your allowed medical absence, your employer is obligated to reinstate you to your previous position or equivalent position at the same pay and with the same benefits. Unfortunately not all employers comply with the requirements of FMLA, and this law will protect you during your breast cancer treatments. If you feel that you have been unfairly treated, you may want to consult an attorney who specializes in employment discrimination issues. At this time in your breast cancer journey, this type of conflict should be avoided if possible and needs to be balanced with your medical care needs. You need to conserve your energy to optimize your medical care and outcome.

CHAPTER 7

Feelings of Being Overwhelmed: Why Me?

Many feelings overwhelm you when you are first diagnosed with breast cancer. The questions you ask during this time, the fear of not making it through, and thoughts of death fill your mind. Feelings of hopelessness and depression also begin to surface while you go through breast cancer treatment. This chapter will help you recognize these feelings and fears and work with the growth that will accompany them. Personal growth is an added-value outcome to facing breast cancer. The opportunity for self-reflection, reassessment of your life values, how you balance your breast cancer experience with your family and work life, and the changes that occur from it, will all be explored.

The Reality Hits: I Have Cancer

You may find yourself walking around at work or at home, or in the car driving and it hits you: I have cancer. The word *cancer* seems to pop into your mind out of nowhere while doing daily activities. At first it may seem surreal and then there is no denying it, you have breast cancer. How do you work with this reality? The word *cancer* constantly flashes like a neon light in your mind and in your world. Allowing breast cancer to be a part of your life without letting it consume your whole life is a difficult task, but it can be done. It takes commitment and purpose. Understand that it has to settle in your mind for a while and you need to not fear your breast cancer, but work with it. In other words, you have to get used to the reality that you have breast cancer. And in some strange way, you become comfortable with breast cancer being a part of your life for now.

In Her Own Words

I think when I was told, I was in shock. I kind of had a bad feeling about the whole situation. I never told anyone until now that I feared years ago that I might get cancer. I don't know why but I did. So when that day came and I was told, I think I thought it was a bad dream.

—Nancy, age 54, 3½-year survivor

Looking at your breast cancer in a detached way may help you accept the reality in order for you to not fear it. You are bigger than your breast cancer. Individuals who can look at themselves from this detached perspective, and even with humor, are recognized as having a healthy survival skill. This technique even has some basis in psychoanalysis—Sigmund Freud used it, theorizing that looking at a problem in a detached way, including with humor, is an effective coping skill when dealing with major life events.

Questioning Your Everyday Life

At times during your breast cancer journey, you look at what is going on around you and wonder why your friends and family are going on with the business of life. Your life as you know it has come to a halt. Those around you are having birthday parties, going to work, going on vacation, and living life as usual. It doesn't make any sense. Feelings of injustice and unfairness begin to take over. You can't understand why your life is not going on as usual. It all doesn't make any sense as you continue to question and try to understand why it feels that you are not fitting in with the world.

In Her Own Words

One thing that I recall from the day my mom was diagnosed is my own thought of losing my own mother at the age of twenty-two. I was so angry that I might not have my own mother around for me when I finally found a great guy and married and had my own children.

—Jennifer Granger, age 26, whose mom is a 3½-year survivor

You ask, do I go on as usual and pretend that having breast cancer is just an added nuisance in my life? Do I put on a happy face for others to make things comfortable for friends and family? How do I fit in with my old life? The answer to these questions lies with you. What you should do for yourself while undergoing breast cancer treatment is your choice. Whatever your choices, it is important to realize that you come first. This may be the first time in your life that you will put yourself first. Women are often the caretakers in the family, the nurturer, and the relationship builders in life. Now, your role must change in order to balance your energy, health, and mental well-being during breast cancer treatment. This is a trial and error approach that is different for each individual. For some women, it may be going on with everyday responsibilities along with your cancer treatments, allowing that sense of "normalcy." For other women, breast cancer treatment makes you question your everyday life and gives you permission to do only those things that work for you. The reality is that the people around you will have to respect what works for you. You may have to help them understand your feelings and in some instances it may not be worth the effort. Breast cancer treatment is at least a six-month to a year commitment and you need all your energy to optimize your health during this time.

The Gloom and Doom Stage

Living with breast cancer brings up the obvious question, "Am I going to make it? Will I live? Will there be life after breast cancer?" It may seem that the only thing that pops up in your mind are thoughts of death and your mortality. You may find yourself preoccupied with death and all things dark. Thinking about your future, your children, your career, and retirement as you did previously is now replaced with thoughts of your life ending. It seems that the people who stand out in your mind are the women who have not survived breast cancer. You may find yourself becoming hypersensitive to all those who have had any type of cancer and paying attention to every detail of their treatment and comparing it to yours.

 Alert

No two occurrences of breast cancer are identical. There are too many variables and unique characteristics of breast cancer tumors, such as size, grade, stage, lymph node status, HER-2 status, along with an individual's wants and needs, that factor into a woman's breast cancer treatment. Also, cancer behaves differently in other body organs and cannot be compared to breast cancer in its treatment and expectations of side effects and outcome of treatment.

No matter what stage of breast cancer you have, you may become preoccupied with death. The outcome of your breast cancer treatment cannot be predicted. Breast cancer is a life-threatening disease and whatever stage you are in, this reality can bring feelings of hopelessness and despair. It is normal for you to experience this overwhelming gloom and doom outlook. Recognizing this as part of the breast cancer experience will help you to not fear the feeling, acknowledge it, and keep your goals of treatment in mind.

Accept Full Responsibility for Your Life

Commit to fighting your breast cancer. Decide how you want to live during your breast cancer treatment and envision health in your future. Accepting full responsibility for your life while on your breast cancer journey means what it says. Having breast cancer requires acceptance, commitment, and a sense of responsibility to do the right thing for yourself.

There are many hard choices and options that come with the diagnosis of breast cancer and it is most likely the first time in your life that you are making choices that have a life and death impact. Taking full responsibility in your course of treatment has very serious connotations. Empowering yourself, learning as much as you can, and knowing how you want to live your life, carries much weight in the balance of staying healthy throughout your breast cancer treatment. Commit to doing the best you can with the information you have by taking full responsibility for your life in sickness and in health. This is one time your decisions rest with you and you will not be able to blame anyone for your choices. Recognize and embrace this responsibility.

 In Her Own Words

When I was first diagnosed with breast cancer, I went into work and sat with a dear old friend who had just started working with me again. When I was telling her about my recent diagnosis, I was saying "Why me?" My friend looked at me and said, "Why not you?" Why are you so different from others to be immune from breast cancer? That statement got me right off the pity pot and the "poor me's" I was going through.

—Theresa, age 46, 4-year survivor

Recognizing Signs and Symptoms of Depression

It is a normal reaction to feel depressed when diagnosed with breast cancer. Feelings of being overwhelmed, anxious, and fearful of the future lend themselves to a feeling of general depression. This is often referred to as reactive depression—depression in response to a life circumstance.

It is an understandable reaction to have feelings of depression when dealing with ongoing breast cancer treatment. Some of the side effects of depression common in cancer treatment include:

- Chronic fatigue
- Sleeping problems
- Changes in eating habits
- Loss of appetite because of medications
- Feelings of hopelessness and uncertainty concerning the outcome of your cancer treatment

 In Her Own Words

To me, the anxiety before any testing or surgery or even chemo has been the most difficult part. The MRI, ultrasounds, biopsy, even surgery weren't so bad because all I really had to do was show up. Hypnosis and meditation beforehand helped me through it all.

—Julie, 28, 2-month survivor

There are usually social workers or nurses where you are receiving your cancer treatment who can offer support. Or they can refer you to a local breast cancer support group. If you are a private person, you may want to seek individual counseling regarding your breast cancer treatment and its impact on your life and feelings. Sorting these feelings out with a professional can make all the difference in your cancer treatment.

The goal is to position yourself with a strategy of health; depression brings down the spirit and will to live. Depression can compromise your immune system at a time when you need to come from a position of strength. To use a football analogy, depression can be the offense and you have to be the defense, ready to tackle it head-on with the support of your team. Remember, depression is not bigger than you and your team. If you have a genetic predisposition to depression or were depressed prior to your diagnosis, then it is recommended that you seek professional help. It will be important to share with your counselor what medications you are taking so they will not interfere with your breast cancer treatment.

In His Own Words

I felt so helpless when my girlfriend was diagnosed, like I'd been punched in the gut. All I felt I could do was go with her to appointments, and after she started chemo, sit with her to watch TV, making sure she's got something to eat and drink and making sure she's comfortable. I realized that just being present means so much.

—Mark, 28, boyfriend of Julie, 28, 2-month survivor

After breast cancer treatment, depression can take you by surprise. You think you should be happy now that your treatment is over. Recognize this as a common occurrence: While you are actively receiving cancer treatment you feel that you are doing something about it and are fighting to eradicate it, but when breast cancer treatment is over, it is hard to rely on your own body to be healthy and not make cancer cells. You feel like you have to gain the trust back that your body will stay healthy. This requires a lot of energy, but if you're aware of it, you can position yourself to be healthy.

Most women who are living with a breast cancer diagnosis feel a sense of sadness and depression at various stages of their treatment. Your life has changed forever and perhaps you have been thrown into early menopause. Your life as you knew it has been turned upside down. Who wouldn't feel sad and depressed at times? Because it is a "normal" occurrence to feel this way when going through breast cancer treatment, the symptoms of a clinical depression may not be recognized by your family, friends, or even health care providers. Depression is a manageable problem that can accompany your breast cancer diagnosis. Here are some signs for you to be aware of that may indicate that you have a clinical depression that may warrant the help of an accredited psychotherapist:

- An inability to cope
- An overwhelming feeling of helplessness and hopelessness
- Inertia (an inability to move or act)
- An inability to concentrate
- Memory problems
- Panic attacks
- Loss of pleasure in what used to make you happy
- Lack of interest in sex or food
- Sleep disturbances

 Fact

If your doctor has prescribed an antidepressant medication, be aware that it may take up to six weeks before you feel its effects.

As you can see, many of these symptoms are common during your course of breast cancer treatment. A good rule of thumb is that if you are having a difficult time moving through these feelings, seek the help of a professional. Sometimes even one visit can make a big difference in how you view the world.

Fear of Recurrence

Once you are diagnosed with breast cancer, your life as you know it is forever changed. Breast cancer treatment seems to take up most of your life while you are going through it. Going to doctor's appointments, follow-up appointments, diagnostic testing, and, after treatment, knowing that you body made the cancer cells that started the whole thing in the first place, may make you feel more vulnerable to getting the breast cancer back. The fear itself can begin to affect you physically and can precipitate the risk of breast cancer's return. Breast cancer is part of you for an entire year, walking beside you as an unwelcome guest. With time, it begins to recede in your mind's eye, but breast cancer is not something you can truly put behind you. Time helps as far as not letting breast cancer define who you are and taking up residence in your mind. Yet fear of recurrence, at some level, is a battle for most women living with breast cancer. The good news is that the longer you do not have a recurrence, the better the odds are that you will not get breast cancer again. Even though most women strive for the five-year guideline to remain cancer-free, biologically speaking, there is no magic five-year milestone. Breast cancer can reoccur many years after the initial diagnosis.

 In Her Own Words

Thinking of the possibility of a recurrence of breast cancer can really get you down if you let it. I have finally figured out that worrying about something that I have little or no control over is just a waste of time that I can spend in more positive ways to keep myself happy and healthy.

—Karleen, age 72, 1½-year survivor

Commit to Growth, Not Perfection

Going through breast cancer treatment is a journey of growth—but it's not one that you would have voluntarily chosen. Having breast cancer subjects you to a new way of life, new concerns, new worries, and new situations. These challenges are what contribute to personal growth in areas that may have been foreign to you before your breast cancer diagnosis. When perfection is your goal, you set yourself up for disappointment. A thinking process that promotes a black and white approach is not constructive. Breast cancer is grey and there is no perfect way to treat it.

Essential

> Breast cancer is actually grey and not black or white. The whole breast cancer experience is many different shades of grey. Personal growth occurs most when you meet life challenges and you learn to cope in a way that works for you.

Keep Your Goals in Mind, Reassess, and Make Changes

Once your decisions are made, it is important to keep your goals in mind and remember what brought you to your decisions. It is best to follow through with your decisions on cancer treatment, whether it is adjuvant chemotherapy treatment or aggressive chemotherapy treatment. You don't want to make a half-hearted decision by starting chemotherapy and deciding against it mid-treatment. However, if you and your oncologist have reassessed your situation and it is determined that a treatment change is appropriate for you, then make the necessary changes.

Visualizing your goals of health and healing is another technique that can help keep you on track. Part of setting goals is first deciding if you want to live and what it is that you want to accomplish in your lifetime. What work needs to be done? You have to ask yourself why you want to live and what is the meaning of you life. This perspective gives you a sense of the meaning of your life, a sense of control in the accomplishments of having future goals. Keep your future goals in mind. Keep your eye on the prize; here the prize is getting through treatment and the hope for wellness and health. It is easy to get discouraged when you are not feeling well from the breast cancer treatments. Chemotherapy and radiation contribute to fatigue, and other side effects that result in a general malaise and loss of energy. It will take all of your energy and purpose to keep your goals in mind. Recognize your life goal, accept your goals of treatment, and work with it as best you can.

CHAPTER 8

Sharing Your Diagnosis

After the shock of hearing the news that you have breast cancer, the next big hurdle that you face is how you tell the people in your life about your diagnosis. You will learn much from others' reaction to the news that you have breast cancer. You will often feel an outpouring of love and support from those that you have confided in and even from acquaintances that know you are undergoing breast cancer treatment. This chapter will give you some guidelines to help you tell those that you have chosen to tell and those who may ask. Most importantly, you will explore how having breast cancer affects your closest relationships as well as your future relationships.

How to Tell People You Have Breast Cancer

In general, there is no right or wrong way to tell people you have breast cancer. Some tips have been identified by experts that can help women who are trying to decide when and how to share the news:

- Take your time. You do not need to tell everyone today or even tomorrow. You may want to wait and plan what you will say when you share the news; just make sure that you feel comfortable when you decide to do so.

- Practice what you are going to say.
- Write down what you want to say.
- Seek out other breast cancer survivors to talk to, and get their advice.
- Take someone with you to help tell your loved ones, if appropriate.
- Be prepared to let them know how they can help, and identify a list of ways they can support you.
- Do less caring for others and more for yourself.
- Tell others when you are ready.
- Focus on getting support and not giving it.
- Consult your physician for more information on how to share the news of your breast cancer diagnosis. Perhaps a joint visit with your doctor will help facilitate the conversation.

People's first reaction is to ask if they can help in any way, so being prepared for this will help you give them some ideas. You know your friends' and family's strengths and what they are capable of giving. Take inventory and, most importantly, let them help you.

In Her Own Words

My sister was diagnosed with breast cancer seventeen years ago. She was thirty-nine years old, my baby sister. I was scared and shocked when she told me. As she shared with me what the doctor told her and how she felt, I knew I needed to be strong and optimistic for her. She is now a survivor and a good friend. I love her.

—Connie, age 73, sister of breast cancer survivor

Telling Your Spouse/Partner

Most often, your spouse/partner knows from the beginning. Open communication with your spouse/partner will be the most helpful to you during breast cancer treatment. You will be experiencing many side effects from breast cancer treatment and many changes in your concept of self, body image, physical changes, and changes in the energy you felt prior to breast cancer. This has a significant impact on your partner, and although you may not feel that he understands your journey, he will be experiencing a parallel journey alongside you.

Expect to feel differences as you go through breast cancer treatment, especially in your body integrity, your energy level, and the appearance of your breast or breasts. Acknowledge the differences, be aware of these feelings, whether of change or loss, so that you can work through these changes yourself. This will help when sharing your feelings with your spouse as your body continues to change and feel different. Be aware that you may be struggling with your new appearance and may be sad that your body does not feel or look the same as it did before your breast cancer treatments. You may be more self-conscious with your loved one about your appearance, or you may notice changes in your sexual health. Open communication with your loved one will promote a safe and comfortable environment to help you be yourself. Discussing changes in your sexual health with your doctor may help you learn about coping strategies to maintain intimacy during breast cancer treatment. Some of the side effects from breast cancer treatment will have an impact on your energy and your ability to maintain good sexual health during and after treatments.

Being Intimate During Treatment

During breast cancer treatments, many of the side effects fight against your desire to be intimate with your partner. As your body is changing, your physical and emotional energy is depleted; your lack of sexual interest seems to take over while you are trying to maintain a sense of normalcy in your life. It feels like you need every ounce of energy that you can muster up just to survive the day. So who is thinking about sex? Most likely, your partner will be. You may find yourself struggling with your own needs and those of your loved one may be the last thing on your mind. The good news is that you, too, will be thinking about your sexual health and needs at various times during your own breast cancer journey. Some women are able to continue with their previous sexual patterns during their treatment while others may find it very difficult. It is important to communicate these feelings to your partner, because he can be of great support to you and help you to feel complete. If you find that your partner is not understanding during this time, you may want to focus on returning to a healthier place in your physical and emotional being before addressing your concerns. You may also want to refer your partner to a support group for guidance and understanding of your support needs so that you do not become *his* support person.

Essential

The loss of libido or sexual desire, whether before or after breast cancer treatment, will vary from individual to individual. The change is most significant when you are premenopausal before treatment and were thrown into an early menopause. Your body feels different and it will take your mind and spirit time to catch up to your new body experience. One of the side effects of being thrust into early menopause can be a loss of interest in sex. Individual or couples counseling may be helpful. Remember, you need to be at peace with your body and with its changes.

Some suggestions that have been made to help with your sexual health are recognizing that your desires and energy may change during breast cancer treatment. Tips that have been shared by health professionals and other women living with breast cancer are the use of vaginal moisturizers or lubricants to lessen discomfort during sexual intercourse. Also, consider talking with your partner about engaging in increased foreplay and experimenting with position changes to see if that will help. Medication can also have a significant impact on your sexual health and desires. You may want to discuss this with your doctor to see if changes in medication can be made.

All in all, it is understandable that as you are facing a life-threatening illness, sex may not be first and foremost on your mind. Helping your partner, who is experiencing his own journey alongside you, through open communication and expressing intimacy in other ways, will sustain and strengthen your relationship. Intimacy is the mainstream of sexual health and is at the core of the human experience. Enjoy it when you and your loved one are ready.

 Fact

Women often have associated the use of tamoxifen as affecting their desire for sex and their loss of libido, because of side effects that include hot flashes and sleep interference. These side effects can lead to a general feeling of fatigue, which is what can affect your interest in sex, but studies show that the drug does not directly affect the libido.

Being Intimate Post-Treatment

When you have completed your breast cancer treatments and some time has gone by, there is the expectation that things will get back to normal. Your sexual health is the most personal and life-changing part of your experience. Your prior physical and emotional health has changed from the experience and it may be difficult for your partner to understand as you move further away from your breast cancer diagnosis and treatment. The old adage that time heals doesn't specify how long it will take, but both partners will at some level struggle with returning to the relationship's previous sexual health. You may discover that you do not have the same desires and your present sexual activity will be different. With breast cancer treatment, many permanent changes occur in the body and you and your loved one may need to adapt to those changes to get to a higher level of intimacy. Touching, rubbing one's feet or back, a quiet walk with your loved one at your favorite place, or a romantic dinner for two may be all you need during those dry spells.

In Her Own Words

It was an early morning call I received from Carol, telling me she wanted to come over to talk with me. I knew then her cancer had come back and she was so scared. It was a little under five years from first onset of breast cancer. At this point, when Carol started her chemo treatments, I would go with her, I never missed one. This was so important to be there for her. I helped, because I would keep talking to her through it all. At one point she said, "Dottie, I know what you're doing," to take her mind off of this whole treatment, because it made her so sick.

—Dottie, age 61, sister

Telling Your Parents, Siblings, and Family

Telling your parents and siblings may be very difficult, especially if your role in the family has been to protect others. Many women have difficulty telling their parents. They may feel that it is not natural to be sick before they are and may not know how to tell them or how they will react. With your siblings, there may be guilt associated with you being the one in your family to have breast cancer and you may be worried about what this information could mean to them, especially if there is a familial or genetic predisposition to your breast cancer scenario.

It may be very overwhelming to tell your extended family of aunts, cousins, and so on that you have breast cancer, especially if you are part of a large family. You may want to assign this responsibility to other family members so as to avoid repeating your story and the emotional energy that is associated with telling. You may decide to tell only your immediate family and tell others when you are ready or if the opportunity arises. Or you may never tell them. The choice is always yours who and when to tell.

In Her Own Words

The first thing I felt was fear, the fear that I would not be around for my children; that I would die and leave them. The hardest thing that I have ever had to do in my life was to tell my sons that I had cancer. But, kids are stronger than you think. They do get through it.

—Debra, age 47, 4-year survivor

Telling Your Children

Experts recommend that the sooner you tell your children that you have breast cancer, the better. Most women don't want to tell their children, because they are afraid that it will be too much of a burden for them and they do not want to distract them from their regular routines of schoolwork or other important activities. Telling your children is important but it is your choice. You should discuss how and when to tell your children with your partner. You may also want to include another family member that your child is close to, for support. Your children may be more comfortable asking questions of a close relative who might alleviate any fears or worries they may have about your cancer.

Why You Might Want to Tell Your Children

Children, when approached in a matter-of-fact and informative way, will be very receptive and look to you for your perceptions of the situation and will use it as their guide. They will take your lead with the information presented to them. Telling them avoids secretiveness about the breast cancer, which would instill a sense of the unknown and fear of what is really happening. Children are very perceptive and know that you are not feeling well, so not talking about your breast cancer may bring on more anxiety and fear. Telling them shows your children that you have confidence in their ability to cope and lessens their feelings of being useless during your breast cancer treatment. Having your breast cancer out in the open will give your children an opportunity to express their feelings of sadness and also a chance to support you and it will make you proud of them. Also, by not telling your children, you risk the possibility that they will find out through others, who may not have the sensitivity or the knowledge of what to say and how to provide the support to your child in the way that you know they need.

In Her Own Words

I told my son that God only gives us what we can handle and that through this journey we would build character. Days later, my son asked, "Do I have enough character yet?"

—Chelsey, age 41, 2-year survivor

When You Should Tell Them

You should tell your children as soon as you are able, but also when the time is right for you. You will want to do it in a calm and quiet environment and not during a hectic time in your family's schedule. You want to be available to them afterward in case they have questions or just want you to be there for them.

What to Tell Them

You should use the word *cancer* and not skirt around the issue or give it another name. Call it what it is so that they will understand. Talk to them in simple language that is age-appropriate. Help your children know what to expect during your breast cancer treatments so they will not be surprised about your lack of energy or your hair loss if you are having chemotherapy. You don't have to tell them everything at once. You can give the information in small doses so that they will not be overwhelmed. If your children cry, let them. Comfort them and let them know that you care and allow them to express their feelings so that they will be able to move on along with you.

 In His Own Words

I remember an almost physical, gut fear for my mom and her health, something akin to a general dread or raw emotion. On the more cerebral side, I remember thinking about what my brother and dad and I would do if she didn't recover. I remember being particularly worried about my dad; how would he cope? What would he do if Mom died? At other times I recall feeling fairly matter of fact. In answer to the question, "What will we do?" I told myself we'd cope. When my self responded, "How?" I told it, "We'll find out when we have to."

—**Casey, son of Ellen, 12-year survivor**

Telling Your Friends

Most women find it easier to tell their friends before telling their close family members. In many cases, friendships are relationships in which you are supportive of each other and have developed strong communication skills. Often you have a long history and have gone through other trying experiences and crisis in your lives and have maintained a healthy bond. Friends can be a great support to you during your treatments and your friends can be a support to each other. Breast cancer is a difficult disease to keep from your friends and telling them will surely be difficult. You will know the best way to tell your friends about your breast cancer and the best time for you to have the conversation with them. Once you begin your breast cancer treatment, you will find that the energy to tell them will be compromised, which makes it best to tell them early on so that they can help and support you during this time. Not all friends are capable of being a support to you, so you choose who, and when, to tell. Your friends will react differently to the news and you may not know what to expect from them when they hear it. For those friends who, based on their reaction to your news, will not be able to support you, kindly thank them and move on to those friends who will be there for you in the ways that you need.

 In Her Own Words

> When I first heard about my friend's diagnosis, I spent a lot of time on the phone with her, day and night. The fear was sitting, waiting like a lion ready to pounce and overtake her. We talked, and we just stayed on the phone, sometimes not saying much. I sat on the floor in my bedroom, not really knowing what to say to her, but knowing I had to stay on the phone.
>
> —Marie, age 54, friend

Be ready to let your friends help you, and identify some ways that they can help you before you tell them the news. If your circle of friends is quite large, you may want to consider writing an e-mail to them letting them know about your diagnosis and that you may not be as available. Explain as much or as little as you are comfortable with. Keep them updated when you want to keep in touch and are feeling up to it. Some women find it difficult to tell their story over and over, so writing an e-mail avoids repeating yourself and helps you to save your energy for getting through treatments and the healing process. You may even consider leaving a voice mail on your answering machine about your progress so that you can pick and choose who you will speak to and when. You may feel like you are not a good friend during your breast cancer treatments. This is truly a time where you need to put yourself first. Your true friends will be there for you at the end of your treatments. If they are not, then they really were not your true friends.

Telling Acquaintances

You may be one of those women who freely tells all to your friends as well as your acquaintances. You may feel freer to discuss your feelings, because you know that there will be no consequences or hurt feelings. Some casual acquaintances may be intrusive and you will need to set limits with them. Whatever the situation, telling others about your breast cancer experience requires much emotional work. Strategizing on what to say, when to say it, and how much to say about your breast cancer experience requires focus and energy, and most often falls into place as you continue along your breast cancer journey.

When telling coworkers, you may be pleasantly surprised at their reactions and willingness to help in the work environment. You will need their support, especially now that you will most likely have to adapt your work schedule around your breast cancer treatments. Initially you may have mixed emotions about sharing such a personal situation with your coworkers and find yourself unable to even face them. You may also feel guilty for not being able to carry your workload during breast cancer treatments. This is understandable, especially in the stressful work environment that exists today. Be patient, be strong, and be the best you can be, which is all that anyone can do. You will find some coworkers more understanding than others. Be thankful for those who are supportive to you and don't focus on those who are not.

Telling Future Mates/Dates

Telling a new relationship about your breast cancer diagnosis brings about feelings of uncertainty and fear that you will not be accepted. You may feel self-conscious about the physical changes in your body and are fearful of rejection once your date or future mate becomes aware of your breast cancer disease and the bodily changes that have occurred throughout your treatments. If this person rejects you, this is not a person that you would want to spend quality time with, so move on and keep your options open and enjoy the dating experience.

If you are single and have had breast cancer, you may find it difficult to tell a date or a new relationship that you are a breast cancer survivor or struggle with when you should tell and how much you should tell about your breast cancer. If you have had a lumpectomy, this may not affect you the same way as telling a potential mate that you have had a mastectomy with reconstructive surgery.

 Fact

There is a practice developed by Dr. Leslie Schover called "mirror therapy" that helps women ease into their prior pattern of sexual activity. She suggests a four-step process: 1, use a full-length mirror in a private area of your home and dress up in your favorite clothes; 2, study yourself in the mirror for fifteen minutes and pick out three things you really like about yourself; 3, then try the same exercise in your lingerie; and 4, take fifteen minutes to look at yourself in the nude, and again, pick out some good points that you are happy with.

Some women struggle with feelings that they may not be desirable to their date. Many women struggle with their body image after breast surgery. It is important to feel comfortable with the changes your body has gone through before sharing this with someone with whom you have a special relationship. It is wise to tell someone before being intimate so that you can prepare yourself and your potential mate. Accepting yourself as you are is really the first step in achieving intimacy with your loved one. Look in the mirror to become familiar with your body and its changes, examine the scars on your chest, and work on getting back a positive view of yourself.

Be good to yourself and buy some fancy lingerie to help you feel that sense of inner beauty in your outward appearance. If you have prosthesis, you may want to keep your clothes on at first and gradually work your way into not needing any coverings or "props." What works for you will work for your partner.

CHAPTER 9

Going Through Treatment

G oing through treatment is a process much the same as the experience of finding out you have breast cancer, discovering what it means, and deciding on options for care. This time the situation becomes more real as you begin your breast cancer treatment and gradually learn to work with the treatments and not against them. This mindset will help with upcoming events, such as deciding whether to buy a wig, a turban, or go bald. It will also help with dealing with fatigue, coping with your loss of energy, and working these new unwelcome things into your life, while stacking the chips in your favor for a healthy lifestyle. Sounds strange but yes, you are going to get through your treatments with style and grace and a new sense of strength.

It's All on Your Head—or Was

With most chemotherapy treatments, hair loss is inevitable. The timing may differ depending on the chemotherapy regime you are on. There are theories that placing cold packs on your head will prevent hair loss. If not losing your hair is important to you and you are willing to try it, go for it. However, it is recommended that you consult your oncologist before engaging in any controversial techniques, because she is your partner in your medical treatment.

The first thing you will need to do is decide what will work for you. Your choices are donning a wig, wearing a turban or hat, wearing a partial wig, or going *au naturel*. That's right; some women may decide to go hairless. The important thing is to do what is right for you. The season in which you are going through treatment may also influence your decision. A wig can keep your head warm during the winter months; wearing stylish hats with your wig may make you feel slightly glamorous. Going hairless may sound good during the summer months, especially if hot flashes are a part of your daily repertoire of side effects. You can experiment with different wigs and hair color. It is really up to you and what will work with your unique personality and style.

How Do You Pick a Wig?

You will most likely pick a wig the same way you pick a new outfit. The wig will be part of you for a period of time and you will want to feel comfortable in it, as with a pair of new eyeglasses, a new bra, or new shoes. However, nothing you purchase will have the same emotional impact as buying a wig because of hair loss from chemotherapy treatments. It will be a new accessory in many ways.

 In Her Own Words

I decided to cut my hair off before it fell out. It was a small way to take back some control in this crazy, chaotic experience. Once I made the decision to cut my hair, I knew I wanted to donate it to Locks of Love. My hairdresser was very supportive and helped me on this leg of the journey. She locked the door of her salon after the last customer left. She, my husband, son, and I gave each other a hug, opened a bottle of wine, made a toast to life, and started cutting. I walked in with long hair and walked out with a buzzcut underneath a gorgeous wig.

—Chelsey, age 41, 2-year survivor

A good time to buy a wig is before you lose your hair. This way you can match your current style and hair color to the wig. It is recommended that you cut your hair short prior to your chemotherapy treatments to help ease the loss of hair in addition to the nuisance of finding hair on your pillow and throughout your home, and in your car and workplace. This too is an individual choice; it may be important to you to keep your hair and its length as long as possible. Your oncologist will be able to give you the percentage of women who lose their hair with your treatment option and the timing of it from past medical experience. Individuals react differently to chemotherapy and you may not fit into the norm. Some chemotherapy regimens lend themselves to a slower hair loss, while others such as doxorubicin (Adriamycin) will cause hair loss after your first or second chemotherapy treatment.

Alert

When cooking over a stove or oven, you need to be careful with your wig, because it is flammable. Especially the human hair wigs. It is always prudent to keep away from open flames. This is another good reason to purchase two wigs, though this is not necessary when caution is taken. You can even get out of cooking if you choose, saying that, after all, you wouldn't want to cause a fire!

Wigs usually cost anywhere from $75 to $300, depending on whether you buy a synthetic fiber or human hair wig. Wigs are usually made of synthetic fibers; however there are human hair wigs, and combination hair/synthetic wigs. Washing a hair/synthetic wig is the same as washing your own hair. You can even use the same shampoo, which may be a comforting smell to you while wearing it. Synthetic wigs will often have recommended solutions to use for washing them, or using Woolite may be suggested. You can dry your wig on a shower head or a Styrofoam head wig holder then style and shape it to suite your individual preference. Your regular hairdresser can also cut and shape it to appear more like your natural hair style.

Wigs, turbans, or hair accessories can help you have a natural look while going through chemotherapy. But all would agree there is nothing natural about breast cancer treatments. Don't be surprised if you find yourself annoyed with society's focus on appearances. Hair product commercials seem to proliferate. It will become clear to you how the focus on outward appearances is promoted by the industry and the media. This often influences our own attitudes about hair, beauty products, and defying the natural progression of aging. When going through breast cancer treatments and living with it, you will learn to put aside the societal undercurrents and get back to the real basics of living and aging as gracefully as you choose.

 In Her Own Words

Being bald gave me strength. Every morning I would stand in the shower and picture myself as an Olympic swimmer, all shaved and slippery and strong, ready to dive in and win that gold medal. And I did win . . . I survived.

—Deirdre, age 47, 3-year survivor

Before buying a wig, you first can ask your oncologist or nurse for recommendations of where to look for a wig. They will refer you to area suppliers of wigs and turbans who know how to work with cancer patients. Most hair dressers are often willing to meet you before or after hours to style your wig. Many of the wig suppliers are also very knowledgeable about other products such as turbans, scarves, and creative ways to use them during chemotherapy treatments. It is advisable to bring someone with you to buy a wig, either a close friend or family member.

Emotionally this is often a difficult process and makes the reality hit home that hair loss is inevitable during chemotherapy. It will be difficult to adjust to wearing your wig and you can expect to feel slightly awkward for the first few days, but this soon goes away. If you continue to feel awkward, you can always go to an alternative by wearing a turban, scarf, or going hairless. The choice is yours.

In Her Own Words

To say the least, losing your hair is difficult. Look at the bright side: no more curling iron, no more blow dryer; you save on the expense of shampoo, conditioner and haircuts, not to mention you do not have to shave your legs or underarms. I decided to remain bald, and did not think twice of what anyone else thought. Each day after work, I would put on my sun hat, put down my convertible top and drive home with a great big smile.

—Suzanne, age 52, 1-year survivor

Consider the process of losing your hair as shedding the old and growing the new during and after treatments—a genesis of new life. Before, your body made cancer cells. Now you are undergoing a process to interfere with their growth and keeping your good cells healthy. It's a new way to look at your hair loss; it is a new chance to start over as if reborn. This requires courage and commitment to change lifestyle patterns, to look again at your old ways and start with a fresh outlook.

Dealing with Fatigue

Feeling tired is a common complaint. But the fatigue that comes from breast cancer treatment is commonly described by women as a tired feeling like one they have never before experienced. It is a chemical, radiating tiredness that feels much different than anything you may have felt before. Fatigue varies for each individual, but it is safe to say that this is one of the major complaints for those receiving radiation and chemotherapy treatments. It truly is a tiredness that is felt at a much deeper level. It is a combination of being physically drained of energy and emotionally and psychologically challenged with the everyday reality of breast cancer treatments.

Balancing your work life and your personal life becomes more difficult in a world that already requires you to multitask in order to get through the day. Now fatigue plays a major role. You have to slow down, prioritize, and perhaps give up many of your day-to-day activities and responsibilities during your breast cancer treatments. It is a temporary problem but offers many challenges to women of all ages.

In order to prioritize, you have to know what is important to you. There is no judgment allowed, but only an identification of how to work with optimizing your time and balancing your personal and work life, whether it is caring for your children or elderly parents, or your volunteer commitments. Saying "no" to your usual activities takes practice and may be difficult, but conserving energy will help you cope with the general loss of energy that accompanies breast cancer treatment.

Recognizing the Role of Energy in Healing

Energy is what makes your body, mind, and spirit connect. This energy is a vital life force that is known by different names in different cultures; in traditional Chinese medicine it is known as *qi* (or *chi*), in Japanese it is known as *ki*, and in Ayurvedic medicine it is referred to as *dosha*. These are all derived from ancient practices and nontraditional medicines used for healing that involve energy flow and self-care guidelines that help a person stay healthy and feel good. Generally these practices recognize that we are all individuals with a unique mind and body. We react differently to our everyday life. It takes a tremendous amount of energy for cells to rejuvenate after radiation and chemotherapy treatments. Looking to these nontraditional methods for help in recovering from cancer treatments has brought these ancient practices into the field of modern medicine.

In His Own Words

One specific thing I did for Julie was I went and bought blank cards and went to my friends and coworkers and had them sign the cards with nice and encouraging things. I believe that kindness is powerful and the kindness of strangers can be even more so. It was nice for me also since I saw how many people that never even met my sister were willing to write a little something for her. I also try to keep the mood light for her. As serious as I know the situation is, I believe it's important and helpful to remember that life is too important to be taken too seriously. Remember to breathe, to relax, and to smile. And laugh. As much as you can. It's good for you.

—Justin, sister of Julie, 28, 2-month survivor

There are two kinds of energy, one that can be measured and one that has not yet been measured. The measurable energy comprises much of the diagnostic testing that is used in breast cancer diagnosis, such as electromagnetic fields using magnetic resonance imaging and radiation therapy. Others are ultraviolet light for treating psoriasis and light therapy for the depression precipitated by the changing seasons and lack of natural light. The energy that has not yet been measured involve the use of complementary therapies such as reiki, yoga, healing touch, acupuncture, meditation, and prayer. This energy medicine is gaining popularity and has begun to be studied for its effects on reducing stress and promoting relaxation. These will be discussed further in Chapter 11.

Often, people define what it means to be happy, healthy, and in balance, as feeling full of energy and life. Maximizing this energy is the goal of energy medicine. It is the life-force energy that makes you feel happy and alive. Ayurveda and Chinese philosophy are about combining wellness, harmony, and spiritual growth. One question that is often asked is, how do you live in balance and maintain an energy flow while going through cancer treatment? Living in balance teaches each of us that we are unique, from the foods we eat, to how we deal with stress and the things we enjoy. Breast cancer treatment zaps much of this energy, but you still have the ability to promote balance, conserve your energy, center yourself in the world, and become a warrior grounded in the earth. It is a process of being at peace with your breast cancer and taking a self-guided approach to achieving a state of health, which often is equated with energy and a feeling of wellness. Energy work can help position you as a mountain unable to be moved, and focus you on the prize of getting through your cancer treatments. Open your heart and mind to energy work and allow it to provide you with a sense of empowerment in the midst of the feelings of help-lessness that often go along with breast cancer treatment.

Cancer and Sexuality

Sexuality is not based on your outward appearance but rather a culmination of your sensual inner being; how you view yourself, your body, and your relationships with your life partner. With breast cancer come many fears, fears that are not based in truth. The important aspect of sexuality is communication with your partner and facing these fears. A partner may have a fear of catching cancer from you, which is not possible. Without open communication, this fear may not surface. Once fears are out in the open, they can be discussed and relieved.

Hair loss in a society that promotes all things physical, particularly the importance of outward appearance, can make the most confident woman feel self-conscious when looking at herself or being seen by a loved one when she has a bald head. Having a mastectomy with or without reconstruction surgery carries an element of uncertainty, including the reaction to the loss as well as the reaction of your partner.

There is also nothing attractive about the nausea and vomiting that often accompany chemotherapy treatment. It is important to be true to yourself during this time and balance your sexual needs with that of your partner. Again, this is an individual experience and your reactions and feelings are yours only and need to be respected by those you love. Resuming sexual activity is a personal choice, including when and how often that happens. Depending on your breast cancer treatment and your options, you should consult your doctor or surgeon about how long you should refrain from sexual intercourse. For example there may be no restrictions if you have had a lumpectomy with radiation or hormonal therapy, as opposed to a more involved treatment course that includes a total mastectomy and reconstruction surgery. Intimacy at all levels is encouraged no matter what breast cancer treatment you are having. Intimacy with your partner can also take forms as simple as holding hands, going for walks, or sharing your innermost concerns and passions.

 Alert

Quality of life issues must play a major role in all decisions involving your breast cancer treatment. Studies have shown that reducing side effects, such as hot flashes, can have a positive impact on quality of life. Some studies have looked into the effect of a serotonin, an up-take inhibitor used in antidepressants, that can alleviate some of the symptoms of estrogen loss along with other techniques previously mentioned to enhance your quality of life.

The other side effect of breast cancer treatment that has an impact on sexuality is early menopause. And taking anti-estrogen drugs such as tamoxifen may cause symptoms related to menopause. The likelihood of going into early menopause depends on the woman's age and the doses used in their chemotherapy treatment. Menopausal symptoms may be annoying but do not impede resuming your previous sexual practices. Managing some of the side effects that are part of the menopause experience can help to alleviate some of these annoyances.

Vaginal dryness and thinning of the vaginal tissue can often interfere with sexual intercourse. This thinning is a result of diminished estrogen in your body from chemotherapy, hormone replacement therapy, or being put into early menopause by your breast cancer treatment. There are many products on the market today. Ask your doctor for recommendations. Products that may be helpful include Replens, which can be used as a daily vaginal moisturizer, or Astroglide, another product that can be used during sexual intercourse. Other options you may want to consider are an estrogen cream or an estrogen ring, which introduces a low level of estrogen directly into the vagina. It is recommended that you talk with your oncologist before you choose any of these options, because there may be unique factors in your breast cancer scenario that your doctor may want to caution you about. Estrogen replacement at any level in a women's life has been a topic of controversy lately among physicians and consumers. Breast cancer certainly puts a different spin on the issue and needs to be part of your decision-making, with an emphasis on the fact that quality of life issues are part of human sexuality.

Why Does Your Body Feel Different?

Whether you are undergoing breast cancer treatment or it is part of your past, expect to worry whenever you have cold symptoms, a headache, or a new pain. The good news is that you will be hyper-vigilant in your care needs once you have breast cancer and this will help in early detection of any future recurrences. However, this hyper-vigilance can also drive you crazy. If you recognize it, accept it and move on. Acceptance of these emotions and fears will help you manage them. The longer you are cancer-free, the easier this will seem, but the reality of the mind-body connection can cause havoc in our bodies.

 Fact

> The term *chemobrain* has recently been coined to describe the effect chemotherapy has on an individual's ability to process information. Loss of memory has also been found in men and women who have had high-dose chemotherapy. This has been recognized as a real side effect and not based on one's emotions or tiredness during breast cancer treatment.

Whether you have had chemotherapy, radiation, lumpectomy, or mastectomy, your body does look and feel different. If you have been thrust into menopause, your body will continue to feel different. Perhaps your energy level is not the same as when you were premenopausal and before cancer treatment. The way you process information may feel different and you may find yourself multitasking with less energy than you had in the past.

Fear of recurrence is usually the predominant factor in jumping to the cancer verdict once you have had cancer. After all, it is natural to feel that your body has failed you once, so why not again? Which disregards your many years of health. This is the "is the glass half-full or half-empty?" philosophy. It is all in how you perceive it. Why not perceive the outcome in your favor?

Feeding Your Body— What Is Right for You

You have heard the phrase "you are what you eat." Current literature supports certain foods as cancer-promoting suspects—in other words there is some sound scientific basis, or that they are proven statistically, to make it easier for cancer to develop. On the other hand, foods that have an anti-inflammatory response are healthier and have anti-cancer properties that stimulate the immune system. It is well-documented that the popular Western diet of fast food and processed food aggravates inflammation.

Vegetables and fruits that are pesticide-free are always good choices and it's also better for the environment when you buy and support local produce. According to the Environmental Working Group, an association that advocates healthier food and a healthier environment (*www.foodnews.org*), fruits such as apples, pears, peaches, strawberries, nectarines, raspberries, and grapes, are more likely to be contaminated with pesticides. The vegetables that are more likely to be contaminated are peppers, celery, green beans, potatoes, spinach, lettuce, cucumbers, squash, and pumpkin. When choosing foods that are more likely to be contaminated, it is recommended that you buy organic. Fruits and vegetables that are less contaminated because of their growing methods are bananas, oranges, pineapple, grapefruit, melons, watermelons, plums, kiwis, blueberries, mangoes, papayas, broccoli, cauliflower, cabbage, mushrooms, asparagus, tomatoes, onions, eggplant, peas, radishes, and avocados.

Alert

Studies demonstrate that cancer feeds on sugar. German biologist Otto Heinrich Warburg won a Nobel prize in medicine for his discovery that malignant tumors are primarily dependent on glucose.

Glucose is a by-product of sugar in the body. Today, people eat too much sugar and white flour, which are foods that are considered high on the glycemic index. Glycemic index foods raise the blood level quickly, which triggers the release of a molecule called IGF (insulin growth factor). IGF stimulates cell growth, which in turn makes all cells grow faster, fostering inflammation and helping tumors grow. Researchers are now studying medicine that will act to reduce insulin peaks and IGF in the blood. You may want to consider changing the way you eat by minimizing high glycemic index foods, such as sugar and high-sugar products such as syrups, white bleached flours, sweetened breakfast cereals, jams and jellies, and sweetened drinks and sodas. On the same theory, you can replace high-glycemic foods with foods that have a low glycemic index, such as natural sugars, agave nectar, mixed whole-grain breads and cereal, lentils, peas, beans, sweet potatoes, fruits, green tea, garlic, onions, and shallots.

Feeding your body in a natural way with foods that help activate your immune system and have anti-inflammatory effects has been found to help the body discourage cancer. Choosing foods that have a low glycemic index—that is, foods that do not promote high blood levels of sugar (glucose)—will inhibit the insulin trigger that promotes cell growth. Knowledge is power. You have the choice to position yourself in an anti-cancer stance and feed your body food that is natural, full of nutrients, and is anti-inflammatory in nature and enhances your immune system. The choice is yours. You can also consult with a nutritionist at your hospital to do a personal assessment of your nutritional needs and a recommended dietary plan during and after your breast cancer treatment.

Vitamins and Health Food

There is much controversy about whether to increase your ingestion of antioxidants during chemotherapy or radiation treatments. Primarily there have been very limited studies about large doses of antioxidants and their protective mechanism on healthy cells. You can ask to see the dietitian at your cancer center for guidance about current research. You may want to consider a vitamin regimen after your breast cancer treatment.

Diana Dyer, a three-time cancer survivor and dietitian, in her book, *A Dietitian's Cancer Story,* shares her personal story of taking vitamins to supplement her diet when her breast cancer treatment was over. She felt she needed that extra boost as a protective mechanism. A summary of her recommendations for vitamins that can assist in healing follows. However, keep in mind that there is no data on the value of supplemental vitamins and their benefits for patients with cancer, though current research is investigating this possibility.

- Multivitamin and mineral supplement with approximately 100 percent of the RDA (recommended daily allowances) and a brand with 10mg or less iron per tablet
- Vitamin C: 250 milligrams once per day
- Vitamin E-200IU: taken once per day, with meal or snack to maximize absorption. A natural (d-alpha) vitamin E with mixed tocopherols is recommended.
- Selenium: 100mcg, from high-selenium grown yeast, once per day
- Calcium: 600–1,200 milligrams per day. For osteoporosis, calcium citrate with additional vitamin D is recommended.
- Echinacea root and herb: 400 milligram capsule to stimulate and nurture your immune system
- Astragalus membranaceus root (Chinese herb): 470 milligram capsules is an immune system modulator, one capsule per day
- Herbal teas: especially astragalus, one cup per day; green tea, two to four cups per day

When choosing your vitamins or herbs, it is recommended that you choose a supplement with USP on the label, which means that certain FDA (Food and Drug Administration) requirements for vitamins and herbs have been met. Check the expiration date and take your vitamin or mineral supplement with food.

A natural alternative to help combat the nausea and vomiting associated with breast cancer treatment is ginger tea. You can make your own by steeping ginger in hot water. Also, chamomile tea is found to help induce sleep, and many other herbal teas add nutritional value to your diet. You can also look into seeing a herbologist to make recommendations for your individual needs, but make sure you seek a reputable one. Most natural health food stores may be able to recommend one, or your local cancer center may know of a herbologist that other cancer patients have used.

CHAPTER 10

Healthy Coping

Coping when facing a life-threatening illness takes both courage and the drive to explore and learn about yourself and strategies that will help you get through treatment. You will need to discover your strengths, what makes you happy, what you like best about yourself, and suggestions on how to grow yourself. There is healthy coping, and then there is not-so-healthy coping. For example, excessive drinking, eating disorders, or any self-destructive behavior can be considered poor coping strategies. This chapter will explore some old and new ways to cope with your breast cancer treatment.

Let Friends and Family Help

Rule number one: friends and family want to help. But they may not know how, so you will need to let them know. Not everyone is comfortable with illness and some may find it hard to extend a hand. But let those who want to help, help. There are many ways people can help you while you are going through breast cancer treatment. It may be something as simple as sending you a card or note with heartfelt concern and thoughts of you. Others may want to help with child care, meal preparation, or providing rides for you or your family. Friends and family want to feel useful and it brings them comfort to be able to help in any way they can. The gift of love and friendship can bring people together to support and surround you during your illness. Afford them this opportunity and it will be a win-win situation.

In His Own Words

I think that shining the light of humor on a difficult situation always helps. Obviously cancer is about as serious as things get, and there are some pretty heavy moments. But treating it as the "c" word and forgetting how to laugh doesn't help. We have a great picture of me, my mom, and my dad all in full "cue-ball" mode and all laughing. I had shaved my head for swimming, my dad was naturally glossy, and Mom was in the middle of chemo, but the picture and the situation it captured were both comical. I think everybody feels better if someone can lighten the mood and try and focus on what's going on in life, not just in illness.

—Casey, son of Ellen, 12-year survivor

It is important to recognize that not all friends and family who want to help you may be of support to you. They may be well-intentioned but can be self-centered and often you will find yourself having to be a support for them rather than the other way around. Choose carefully who you let into your circle of support. Allow the ones you can count on to bring you comfort and help lighten your burden. It will make all the difference in the world to you and to your circle of support.

Past Coping Patterns—What Worked?

Examining and identifying what helped you cope during other stressful times in your life can be applied to the problem you have now—coping with the diagnosis of breast cancer and its treatment. Some coping strategies you may have used in the past could include having tea or coffee with a friend you trust or going to the movies or theater to distract yourself from your current situation. Participating in your usual routines can also help during this time.

 In Her Own Words

Partway through my treatment, my oncologist said he was worried about me. When asked why, he said, "Because you are handling this too well." My response to him was that I have breast cancer, but it is not going to get me. I couldn't change what had happened to me, so I chose to make the best of it and go on from there. I strongly feel that a positive attitude will help for a much faster recovery. I am happy to say that eleven years later, even though I deal with ongoing lymphedema, I am still enjoying every day with a smile.

—Diane, age 62, 11-year survivor

Studies have shown that people who keep engaging in new activities, hobbies, and developing themselves, adjust better to illness and stressors and become more resilient and live longer. Some of the reasoning of this theory is that a person tends to use different parts of the brain, and keeping active physically and mentally stimulates the immune system and a general sense of well-being.

Other people who are experiencing the same challenges can also be a support to you while you undergo breast cancer treatment and can be an important part of the healing journey. Seeking out help is always more useful than turning inward, where coping is self-limiting. If being with children brings you joy and lightens your heart, then you may want to schedule time to be with children. Whatever you choose to do, you need to keep in mind that you should balance your "coping times" with times when you are feeling well. You may feel better right before your next chemotherapy treatment is due and your blood counts are up. Also, you need to limit your contact with others who have cold symptoms or other illnesses at this time because your immune system is compromised during breast cancer treatment.

Loss Is the Overriding Theme

When diagnosed with breast cancer, besides being overwhelmed, there are feelings of loss and grief. What happens after diagnosis is that what your old world consisted of—your day-to-day life, concerns, anxieties and goals—seems to be lost. A whole new world of medical interventions and dealing with breast cancer treatment options is your primary focus. Your body image as you once knew it changes, and what was once taken for granted becomes the center of the new life that develops.

There are new concerns and fears about things like losing one's hair and one's breast. Changes and losses that occur, including the possibility of early menopause and the loss of child bearing, which may have a profound impact on the life of a young woman undergoing breast cancer treatment. Feelings of a general loss of control of your health, fears about survival, and lost confidence in your body to fight off disease bring you to a place you have never been. This vulnerable place can be used to strategically put you on the offense. Knowing and recognizing the overriding theme of loss in your life now that you are being treated for breast cancer can help you place yourself in a position of strength. Think of yourself as a mountain, scarred and battered, but unmoved and standing proud. You should allow yourself to experience these feelings of loss and grief to assist you in the grieving process, but then set your mind to overcome them and move forward toward a new life.

Do What You Enjoy Best

Doing what you enjoy best may never be as hard as it is for you when you are going through breast cancer treatments. It may be difficult to identify your sources of enjoyment once your life has been changed by your diagnosis. Your treatments may put a temporary halt to your favorite activities. For example you may be an active person who works out three to five times a week at a local gym. But the side effects of cancer treatments may force you to contemplate a slightly different path, such as yoga or Pilates, which will be discussed in Chapter 11. Discovering new ways to exercise your body and mind with meditation, walking in a local park, enjoying nature, going to the beach, swimming, or golfing all can be part of your recovery as long as you are mindful of your limitations and seek medical advice if you have any concerns. The medical profession recognizes the power of how doing the things you most enjoy may stimulate the immune system and often recommends that you incorporate them into your breast cancer treatment. It is healthy to participate in those things that bring you the most joy during your treatments. Actively seek opportunities to do what you enjoy most. It will benefit your breast cancer treatment as well as your general sense of well-being and health during treatment.

Seek Out Humor

The Proverbs say "a merry heart doeth good like a medicine." And, in truth, laughter brings feelings of well-being and is likened to medicine for the spirit. Norman Cousins in his 1979 book *Anatomy of an Illness* brought the healing nature of humor to the public. Suffering from a collagen disease, his approach was to take large amounts of vitamin C and surround himself with laughter. He was a pioneer in the humor therapy movement. Studies have shown that belly laughing releases endorphins that act as a pain medicine and give the laugher a general sense of well-being. This feeling is very similar to that high one feels after exercising. Seeking out humor and laughing at yourself—for example, putting your wig on a child or a pet—can bring on an old-fashioned belly laugh. This lightens the mood and your spirits, and promotes an environment of healing.

Norman Cousins healed himself not in a hospital environment—he felt this was not an environment that promoted health—but in a hotel room, where he watched funny movies. This is not to say that you can omit your medical treatment, but you can use laughter to enhance an atmosphere of healing and well-being.

In Her Own Words

When a favorite relative of mine was diagnosed, I prayed, sent her funny cards and trinkets faithfully, prayed harder, and found ways for all of us to laugh. Cancer should never be allowed to rob anyone of the privilege of laughter.

—Linda, age 55, relative

Different people perceive humor and what is funny to them very differently. You know what brings a smile to your face and what you need to do to foster those situations of lightheartedness. You can watch movies, listen to happy music, laugh with friends, and share the "funny-scared moments" of your life with breast cancer with others. Finding humor in all you do is a healthy coping strategy. The next time someone tells you that you look great, you could say, "Thank you, but I am having a bad wig day," and watch her expression. Often others are uncomfortable, and don't know what to say, but by you setting the stage with open communication it can make a big difference for yourself and others. The important thing is to find what makes you laugh and make it your business to seek it out. Humor is good for the soul.

Try Journaling

Keeping a journal helps you express yourself, your inner feelings, and fears in a safe environment. Journal writing can be a source of healing and strength while you go through the breast cancer journey. There is no right or wrong way to keep a journal. Expressing yourself in writing helps to identify what you are feeling. This self-awareness helps to clarify your thoughts. As you travel the journey of breast cancer, you are bombarded with many feelings, fears, and concerns. Keeping a journal can not only be enlightening, but can awaken your creative ability. Ira Progoff's book, *At a Journal Workshop,* explains his method as a process of self-discovery and recognition that comes by beginning to reflect on the stepping stones in life. The events that have shaped a person's life so far are the stepping stones. You can call upon journal writing at a time of crisis, but it is available to you at all times in the life cycle. Journaling during breast cancer treatment or joining a writing group with other survivors can be a support to you that travels with you along the way. Your journal will hold in sacred trust your feelings, fears, hopes, and life experiences. Journaling is a self-healing process and spiritual journey as you go through breast cancer treatment.

Journal writing begins at different places for each person who travels the breast cancer journey. Your journal can begin with the discovery, the diagnosis, or the waiting period. You can write about your daily travels, the events of the day, and the feelings that accompany them. You can write about the friends, family, and health-care providers who are your supports along the way. Journal writing can help you express how you are feeling about what is happening to and in your body, including concerns regarding sexuality, hair loss, and fatigue symptoms. As you go through your experiences and process your thoughts and feelings through journal writing, you learn about yourself, your beliefs, and your inner resources. This recognition empowers you through your breast cancer treatment and adds clarity and depth to your experience.

Be Kind to Yourself

Often it is easier to be kind to others, and cut them slack, than it is to do this for yourself. People tend to be harder on themselves than on others. In order to counteract the human inclination of being hard on yourself, you need to vow in your mind and heart to be good to yourself. For example, simply allow yourself the time to go for a walk with a friend or someone who gives you comfort. At this time you may choose to be only with people who bring you up and avoid those who make you feel uneasy about yourself and your breast cancer treatment.

This takes training and effort. For most people time is taken up by the many "shoulds" in life. They may include taking care of others, children, parents, spouses, friends, and partners along with everyday work and household responsibilities. Breast cancer treatment cannot be just added to an already busy life: Prioritize and give up some of your other responsibilities as part of your survival. Feelings of guilt often interfere with the concept of being kind to yourself. For now, you need to give up guilt and start caring about and being kind to yourself.

Join a Support Group

Studies have shown that women who are involved in a support group while going through breast cancer treatment actually do better and survival rates for them are longer than they are for those who do not participate. It is thought that being with others and experiencing the support stimulates a participant's immune system. Being with others who share the experience is a helpful way to deal with the emotional upheaval and issues that occur with breast cancer treatment. When you attend a support group, you will be exposed to other women who are at different stages of their breast cancer treatment. When someone going through treatment is introduced to long-term survivors, it can give her a sense of hope. And when those who may be at the same treatment stage can spend time with each other, they can share experiences and be of support to each other. You will find yourself bonding with certain women in your support group more than others, but in general it is a safe place where you can express your feelings, concerns, and fears without burdening those who are close to you. Breast cancer affects the entire family system and often it is difficult to share with close family and friends, because the experience is not something that they can understand completely as other women living with breast cancer. The breast cancer journey is uniquely yours and what helps and supports you during this time is yours to determine and act on.

 In Her Own Words

> I was fortunate to have found a support group shortly after I was diagnosed in September 2003. I had a lumpectomy, chemotherapy, and radiation as treatment. The whole ball of wax, as they say. My mother was in a nursing home with Alzheimer's and I have no siblings and was living alone with few friends in the area, so the support group became very important to me. I continue to go because I feel it is a way to "give back." I had two friends die of breast cancer and I needed to see that there were survivors. The support group gave me that opportunity.
>
> —**Bevlynn, age 62, 5-year survivor**

Breast cancer support groups have many advantages, and being with others and the friendships that occur are often very healing and empowering. Support groups may not be for everyone, but the important thing is that you have a safe environment to express your feelings and concerns. Individual counseling can also be effective and breast cancer treatment centers usually have social workers you can speak to or who can refer you to a counselor in your area.

Exercise

How you exercised before being diagnosed with breast cancer can set the stage for your continued recovery. If you were active and exercised regularly, you may feel frustrated by your low energy level during your treatments. Adapting your previous level of exercise in your life may be challenging, but also can introduce you to many other forms of exercise, many of which will be discussed in Chapter 11. Maintaining your exercise routine is very important during breast cancer treatment as long as it is tempered to meet your physical needs and your energy level. It is also important to ask your oncologist what is recommended for your specific situation. For example, if you have had a bilateral mastectomy with reconstruction, you will have to follow your surgeon's advice and recommendations on how to exercise.

 In Her Own Words

Energy is diminished with surgery, chemo, and/or radiation, so modify your normal exercise routine. Surgery can take a toll, so I hired a personal trainer who had experience with breast cancer patients and we worked on strength training for the chest and arms. I didn't have energy to run, but walking in the fresh air helped both physically and emotionally.

—Nanci, age 55, 1-year survivor

Your daily exercise routine has a big impact on your sense of normalcy and feelings of well-being, so it is encouraged by health care professionals. The benefits of exercise, whether running, walking, or lifting weights, are well documented. Endorphins that are released with exercise bring a feeling of elation. In breast cancer treatment, you may need to adapt your previous exercise routine temporarily and enjoy being introduced to some alternative modes of exercising your mind, body, and spirit.

Grow Yourself

Getting back to nature or basics promotes growth. It is one of life's forces. Nature teaches us many things, including seeding, growth, and life cycles. All experiences in life promote an inner growth, a journey that is uniquely yours. Personal growth during your breast cancer treatment is a "value-added" side effect of breast cancer treatments. The experience brings you to a new depth of self and your relationships with others. A newfound empowerment and strength may find you in a better place with yourself and others through your breast cancer journey. Being open to new experiences and looking within yourself to get through cancer treatments can open up a new world of adventure. For example, getting a dog this may not have fit into your busy schedule prior to your diagnosis, but now may be an opportunity to bring you much joy as you go through breast cancer treatments and beyond. Whatever brings you new joy and peace that you have discovered through your breast cancer journey can be yours to keep and enjoy.

CHAPTER 11

Exploring the World of Complementary Therapies

Complementary therapies are not meant to take the place of traditional treatment options, but should be used as a complement to traditional therapies, to control symptoms and side effects, and to promote a sense of well-being during breast cancer treatment. Exploring the many options—such as meditation, yoga, Pilates, reiki, massage, acupuncture, Healing Touch, art therapy, and diet—can help with your breast cancer treatment by managing its side effects as well as discovering new ways to manage stress. Finding harmony, peace, and balance during cancer treatment can pave the way for a healing journey that relieves stress and enhances your quality of life both during and after breast cancer treatment.

Meditation

Meditation practices have been used for many thousands of years. One method that is used often in breast cancer treatments is called mindfulness meditation. This is a simple way of focusing your mind and thoughts on the present moment. The goal of mindfulness meditation is to be aware of what is happening in the present moment. Most often, people are in a more reactive mode, responding to the environment, being lost in thought, whereas with mindfulness meditation the focus is on the moment. Mindful meditation is about rediscovering the present moment. Often, meditation practices can help manage the many side effects of chemotherapy and radiation and promote a sense of wholeness. When you are in the present and aware of your surroundings, you are more connected with yourself. With daily practice, you can benefit from living in the moment and fully experiencing the here-and-now. The present moment is all you really have. And you are alive to grow, discover, learn, and "be" within it, so that you can find a sense of balance and express the emotions that you are experiencing.

Being present in the moment helps to create a series of special moments, because you are alive and awake in it. What is most important to cultivating this mindfulness is to make the time in your day for fifteen to twenty minutes to meditate. You can get up earlier in the morning and begin incorporating it into your usual morning activities.

Essential

There are many forms of meditation; they can be structured or unstructured. But most will help ground you in the practice of living in the moment and enjoying the present, so that you will be free to embrace life more fully and empower your mind to be focused and open to new adventures even while you go through breast cancer treatment.

Meditation involves a nonjudgmental attitude toward your thoughts and helps to keep your thoughts focused. When meditating, your thoughts may wander to events of the day or what needs to be done, but you can teach yourself to gently return to focusing on your breath and your meditation. Meditation helps you allow things to be as they are and you can learn to "be" with whatever comes to your heart and mind. Of all the complementary methods, meditation is the easiest to begin during breast cancer treatment. You can do this at home with very little instruction. Here are some basics to get you started.

Posture

It is best if you can sit on a cushion, either on the floor or in a chair, with your back straight. If you are sitting in a chair, let both of your feet touch the floor. The hands may rest in your lap or be placed on your thighs. Imagine yourself sitting in a relaxed place.

Begin to Meditate

You can begin just by being aware of the fact that you are sitting. You can begin at your feet and toes and go up through your legs, pelvis, abdomen, chest, heart, shoulders, arms, hands, neck, and head, being aware of how they are feeling in your body. Start with your toes, feel the weight where they touch the floor, experience an awareness of your body and then go gently up your body with a heightened awareness of how it feels to be present and aware of yourself. Allow yourself to settle into your body and into the moment. Closing your eyes may help you to focus or pick a spot on the floor in front of you where you can rest your eyes.

Focusing on the Breath

Gently bring your awareness to your breathing, the gentle rising and falling of your belly. Notice each detail of the experience of breathing, when it is the strongest for you. Focus on the "rising and falling" of your belly as it lifts as you inhale and falls as you exhale.

Gently Working with the Mind

You will probably be aware of your thoughts interfering with your concentration and, before you realize it, you are no longer focused. Recognizing that stray thoughts will enter your mind is normal, but you need to gently return to your breathing exercise to begin again. This is part of your meditation practice and the more you practice, the easier you will find it to maintain your focus. Remember to be gentle with yourself throughout the meditation process.

Yoga

Yoga offers relief from the side effects of treatment for many women with breast cancer. Yoga helps to promote a feeling of well-being and balance, which helps a person experience a wholeness of body and spirit. Many losses are likely to occur during breast cancer treatment—loss of appetite, hair, body image, and energy—and many women are finding this ancient discipline can comfort and help them feel whole again. Yoga often helps reduce breast cancer treatments' side effects. Studies suggest that doing yoga while going through treatment helps the patient get through it with fewer side effects by reviving her sense of energy and making her feel good mentally. Other research has shown that yoga can ease the nausea, depression, and anxiety that often come with breast cancer treatments.

Yoga can be done in a class setting or in your home. With regular yoga practice, you will get a sense of physical movement and experience peace, harmony, and inner strength. Through yoga, you will feel the benefits of exercise while balancing your breast cancer treatments, providing you with techniques that promote healing and reduce anxiety.

 Fact

Yoga practice can be a helpful tool to see you through breast cancer treatment, as noted in an October 2008 *Yoga Journal* article written by Katherine Griffin. Special yoga classes for breast cancer survivors are offered at many cancer centers. You can also join a yoga class in your area and tell your instructor about your special needs during your cancer treatment. Always consult your doctor prior to participating in yoga classes.

Jinani Chapman, a yoga teacher and registered nurse who works with cancer and chronically ill patients at the University of California-San Francisco's Osher Center for Integrative Medicine, developed six poses to see you through treatment. They are reprinted here with her permission. The poses were designed to help with lymph drainage and for anyone in treatment for breast cancer, but can also be used in all stages and treatment of breast cancer. It is recommended that you consult your health-care provider and team to get their approval before you undertake this type of physical activity.

The Hip Walk

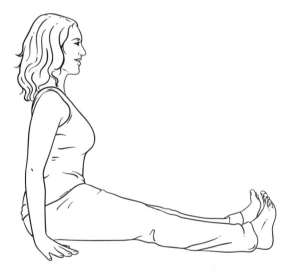

This pose is designed to boost energy, activate pelvic and abdominal muscles, and massage organs, along with promoting lymph drainage.

Begin by sitting erect on the floor with your legs extended in front of you. As you inhale, consciously elongate your spine upward through the crown of your head so that the pelvis tilts slightly forward and the back is straight. Alternate scooting or lifting first one hip and then the other forward until you have moved to the front edge of your mat. Then walk your hips backward in the same way. Continue "walking" forward and backward for a few minutes or as long as it feels comfortable. Use deep breaths and abdominal contraction on exhalation.

The Cormorant

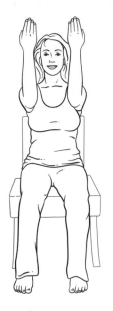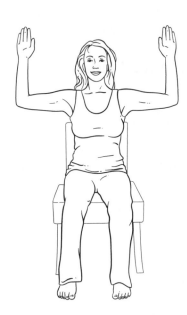

This pose helps activate and strengthen the midriff and chest muscles by promoting healing after lymph node dissection.

Begin by sitting on a chair with both arms extended out in front of you parallel to the floor or at a slightly higher angle. Bend your elbows to 90 degrees. Throughout the movement, keep the lower arms perpendicular to the floor and parallel to each other, with each hand directly above its respective elbow. Keeping the arms and elbows at shoulder height or slightly higher when moving them allows gravity to facilitate lymph drainage down the arms and into the chest. Exhale as you bring the elbows toward each other in front of you. Be sure to keep the forearms parallel to each other—do not let the hands come any closer to each other than the elbows are able to come. Then, inhale and fill your lungs to capacity to open the chest upward as you open the arms as far out to each side as they'll go. Maintain each hand directly above each elbow. Continue this practice for as long as it feels comfortable. Start small, with a few repetitions; you can build to eight or ten repetitions over the course of a few weeks. Rest as needed.

The Silly Teapot

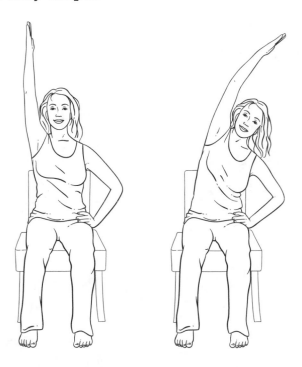

This pose helps to activate the inner and outer intercostal muscles (the rib muscles) to deepen breathing and stimulate the flow of lymph fluid through the trunk of the body and through the arms.

Sit on an armless chair and place your left hand on your left hip for support when you start moving. Imagine that your torso is a teapot that you are filling as you inhale. Lengthen the spine upward from the tailbone to the crown of the head. Lift the right arm alongside your right ear, pointing the hand toward the ceiling (or bend your right elbow and cup the back of your head with your hand). On an exhalation, bend sideways to the left in a flat plane. Imagine that you are pouring the tea out through the right hand or elbow. Keep your chest open and your shoulders stacked (no twisting or turning) as you tilt sideways, with both sides of the torso long. Return to the vertical position on the inhalation. Repeat the same movement on the other side.

The Cat Purrs

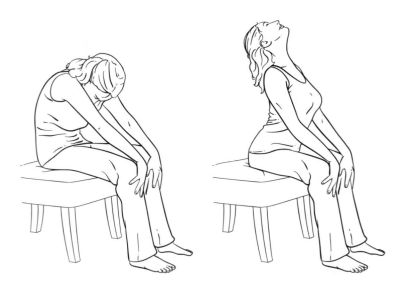

This pose is found to increase spinal flexibility, and encourage abdominal strength.

Sit erect and comfortable on the front edge of your chair with your feet on the floor or supported by a cushion. Place your palms on your knees. Exhale as you tuck in your tailbone and point it forward to round your pelvis and lower back. Continue rounding along the entire spine and tuck your chin toward your chest as you extend your arms forward on the thighs. Then, inhale as you point your tailbone down toward the floor, drawing your hands up along your thighs. Elongate up through the spine to a gentle arch. Lift the chest upward. Exhale each time you tuck and round; inhale each time you extend and elongate. Remember to purr as you relax into the movements of this sequence, enjoying whatever range of motion you have along the forward and backward axis of the spine. Witness how you feel as you explore your range of movement vertebra to vertebra.

The Winding Twist

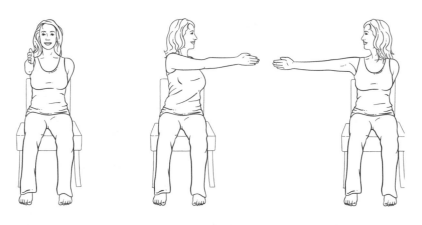

This pose stimulates the muscles along the spine and massages the internal organs.

Stay seated in your chair, lengthen your spine, and reach the crown of your head toward the sky. Rest your feet on the floor, with each knee directly above each ankle. Place your left hand behind you, palm down on the chair seat, and extend the right arm out in front of you, parallel to the floor. Follow that hand with your gaze as you exhale and twist to the left, palm facing left, for the base of the spine. Invite that right arm to stay parallel to the floor. Time your exhalation to finish when you reach the full range of your twist. Then inhale as your right arm returns, with the palm turned in the direction of the movement. As you continue inhaling, let the arm sweep around to the right side of the body. Continue coordinating the breath with the movement and rest at the first sign of tiredness or muscle fatigue. Switch sides and continue for as long as comfortable.

The Settling Self

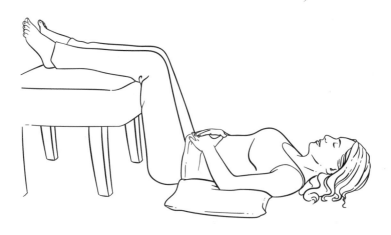

This pose uses gravity to help the lymph fluids drain toward the front of the chest. This helps circulation and lymph node drainage and calms and balances the nervous system, which in turn settles the mind.

Lie on your back on a cushioned mat and rest your calves on a chair at a height that allows your knees to be at a 90-degree angle.

Rest your arms away from your torso, off to the sides, elbows slightly elevated on soft pillows, and place your hands on your abdomen. You can let the eyes close or use an eye pillow if that feels comfortable. Exhale and draw your abdominal muscles toward the spine as you breathe, and imagine the energy generated from your practice flowing through your palms to nourish your center. Reflect on the miracle of being alive and invite your conscious imagination to direct healing energy through the breath to every cell, every muscle, every tissue, every organ, and every system in the body so that you are envisioning physical, mental, emotional, and energetic healing. Rest here in the center of your being, restoring and renewing the life within you.

Pilates

As in yoga, in Pilates you engage your body and mind in a series of precise, focused exercises. Joseph Pilates, who developed the method, was a sickly child. He became a physical trainer and explored yoga, gymnastics, skiing, dance, weight training, and other therapeutic regimens.

Because of its low-impact nature, you may feel that you are getting very little benefit from it, but Pilates teaches you to retrain your body and strengthen its core by a total body-conditioning workout. Pilates focuses on a properly aligned body, balanced and graceful, that promotes good habits that will help keep your body strong.

The benefits of Pilates are that it tones muscles and improves posture. It is low impact and can help prevent injuries in dancers and athletes and can even help heal injuries when used as a therapy. It is also known to boost the immune system, increase bone density, and make your joints more limber and your body more flexible. The practice of Pilates also focuses on breathing to reduce stress and leaves you with a feeling of being re-energized. When undergoing breast cancer treatment, capitalizing on conserving energy and strengthening your inner core helps to assist in the healing process.

One of the basic principles of Pilates is breath. It uses a breathing technique called lateral breathing, in which inhalation is a preparation for starting a movement, while exhalation accompanies each movement. You should also always remember to keep breathing throughout the movement and not hold your breath. Concentration is needed and engaging the mind in thinking about moving is the only way to do Pilates properly. This technique is helpful with all activities of life. It gives you greater clarity and reduces stress. Pilates is about mastering your mind and doing things slowly and measurably, keeping your movements in control.

Essential

Pilates was once used primarily by dancers, actors, and celebrities, but in the 1990s as high-impact aerobic exercise programs decreased in popularity, Pilates gained widespread recognition. Pilates uses many techniques to achieve its goal of body core work. There are usually several options, such as mat work, individual instruction, and use of specialized machines, such as the reformer, the Cadillac, the wunda chair, and the magic circle (which helps with flexibility and stability).

Being centered in Pilates means two things. It means being able to remain steady and balanced with good posture. It also means engaging the center of your body, your core muscles that go around your body from just below your ribs to the tops of your legs. To see results, quality (not quantity of) movements, and proper alignment are emphasized. Going with the flow, connecting movements that are harmonious and graceful, makes Pilates a useful complementary method during breast cancer treatments, depending on what your interests and needs are. If you are looking for a fitness program that you can do while going through breast cancer treatment that strengthens your core muscles and improves body alignment, Pilates might help you achieve your goal. Whatever your goals are, it is important to check with your health care team and doctor to make sure that this is a viable option for you and that your doctor agrees before you embark on a Pilates regimen.

Reiki

Reiki is a Japanese word meaning "universal life energy." It is a gentle method of hands-on healing that taps into one's energy. It is referred to as *ki* in Japanese, *chi* in Chinese, and *prana* in Indian. Reiki is not massage, hypnosis, or a tool for diagnosing illness, but rather a technique that uses energy flow to promote balance of body and mind. Reiki can alleviate pain and stress and promote restful sleep, healing, and relaxation. Reiki is a gentle art that draws on universal life energy to benefit women who are in breast cancer treatment. This philosophy of health and illness comes from ancient Buddhist healing arts, which operates from the belief that illness is caused by energy that is blocked in the body. Reiki helps restore the flow of energy, to balance and harmony in the body.

 In Her Own Words

Reiki is energy work that reduces stress and promotes relaxation to allow the body to heal itself. IET (integrated energy therapy) releases the blockage in the tissues that can cause pain or discomfort. These energy modalities are wonderful. I have been a Reiki/IET practitioner for several years and have used this work on a regular basis. It helped with the nausea, bone pain, and overall anxiety that I felt during chemotherapy treatment and follow-up testing. And I am still using the energy work every day.

—Suzanne, age 43, 3-year survivor

To receive Reiki, most people lie on a table fully dressed. It is important to wear comfortable clothes, even though little or no pressure is applied. The technique can also be done in a chair or hospital bed. The Reiki practitioner is focused and centered on the energy that flows through the practitioner to the subject. You will receive the amount of energy that you need to feel balanced, nurtured, and cared for. Usually a deep sense of relaxation, calm, and well-being occurs as a result of Reiki energy.

Research on various types of energy work has shown that Reiki not only brings a deep sense of relaxation, but also promotes a decrease in anxiety, pain, and muscle tension. It can also facilitate wound healing and enhance a feeling of wellness and a general sense of health.

Massage

Massage is another nonpharmaceutical technique that uses hands-on touching to move the soft tissues of the body. There are different forms and levels of pressure and touch used in massage. It can be more of a superficial pressure on the skin or the pressure can go deep into the underlying muscle tissue.

Alert

Most massage includes the use of oils or lotions on your skin, so if you are especially sensitive to these, you need to tell your massage therapist. Also, if the pressure used is too hard and you are uncomfortable you need to tell your massage therapist.

The major benefit of massage is to relieve pain, anxiety, and fatigue. Massage also relaxes the muscles and has been known to stimulate the immune system. It is important to tell your massage therapist about your breast cancer treatment so that she can adapt the massage to your needs and avoid areas that may be sensitive. A typical massage can last anywhere from thirty to ninety minutes. There are shorter massage techniques, such as hand and foot massage that can be done during chemotherapy treatments. Some cancer centers offer these services to help relax and enhance a feeling of wellness.

When choosing a massage therapist, you should ask about her training, background, and if she has worked with cancer patients before. It is important to find out if the massage therapist is licensed or certified. There are state-by-state requirements for education and experience, so it is recommended that you check on the training and certification of the masseuse in the state in which she is practicing. The American Massage Therapy Association and the National Certification Board for Therapeutic Massage and Bodywork are organizations that provide information about massage therapists in your area and their credentials. You can always ask your surgeon or oncologist for their recommendations.

Some basic guidelines when having massage therapy are to avoid deep massage during chemotherapy and radiation therapy. Chemotherapy and radiation therapy already put extra strain on your body and massage should promote relaxation and comfort, not cause more pain and discomfort. Avoiding sensitive areas or using light touch massage post-surgery, especially if you have had total lymph node dissection or experience lymphedema, is important. Also, if you have markings on your chest and arms for radiation therapy, it is advisable to avoid oils and lotions on these areas.

Overall, massage therapy offers an alternative technique that has been found to promote relaxation, and decrease anxiety, pain, and depression. Physically, studies have actually shown an increase in the level of dopamine, which helps provide a feeling of well-being, after having massage therapy.

Acupuncture

Acupuncture, a Chinese form of medicine, involves the five elements of hope, compassion, service, forgiveness, and courage. All these things make up the spirit, which is considered the most important essence of who you are and your unique presence in the world. In traditional Chinese medicine (TCM), acupuncture is considered one of the techniques that can benefit people with cancer. Acupuncture is based on the theory that there are meridians or channels of energy (chi) that flow through your body.

 In Her Own Words

I didn't believe that reiki or acupuncture would work on my pain and growing anxiety. Then one morning as I plugged in my hair dryer I realized I didn't "believe" in electricity either, but it worked. So I plugged myself into treatment and found that it was just what I needed. Every Saturday I felt cared for, safe, and relaxed.

—Deirdre, age 47, 3-year survivor

In acupuncture, fine needles are inserted into the skin at specific points in order to move energy around or unblock areas that may be cluttered or stagnant, and thereby causing illness. Integrating TCM may ease breast cancer side effects by working on those points that are identified to restore your balance and energy flow and promote healing and an overall feeling of well-being. Energy (chi) blockages are thought to be caused by many sources such as diet, genetics, history, exercise, work, environment, and lifestyle activity. Blockage of chi, according to TCM philosophy, is what leads to illness and cancer. Also, stress and depression can affect energy flow, so that the interconnectedness of energy, body, mind, and spirit influences our reactions. Acupuncture can help balance our reactions and energy flow and may be useful in restoring harmony.

Healing Touch

Healing Touch therapy is a noninvasive complementary method of treatment that uses light touch with the hands to move the energy flow within the body. Unlike massage, Healing Touch often does not touch the body but uses energy and only light touch to improve health and balance.

Healing Touch manipulates energy fields around the body and supports the body's ability to heal with the goal of increasing a sense of well-being. Healing Touch is a nursing intervention, and was actually pioneered by nurse Janet Meutgen. It combines energy and touch to minister to the energy system that can be disrupted by illness, disease, stress, and surgery.

Healing Touch interventions have been found to have a profound effect on the relaxation response and enhance mood. Many nurses use Healing Touch in the health care setting to help reduce pain and anxiety, assist in wound healing, reduce side effects of chemotherapy and radiation, and normalize blood pressure. Healing Touch involves electromagnetic energy fields, the life flow, chi, and the energy around the body known as the aura. There has been some research on the therapeutic effects of Healing Touch in managing cancer treatment side effects, such as nausea and fatigue. Most studies look at a patient's perceptions of their feelings of well-being before and after treatment and the procedure's effect on the immune system. Although the beneficial results of Healing Touch are not fully understood, there are studies underway to measure its effects on energy, healing, and balance.

Art Therapy

Art therapy is a complementary therapy that helps a person express herself creatively in a safe environment. Creating art has been found to improve a person's sense of physical, mental, and emotional well-being. The ability of a person to express herself in positive ways has an impact on her self-esteem, and therefore helps improve her overall health. Through creativity, art therapy can help you to express your pain and fear in a safe venue.

Much of the therapeutic benefits of art therapy come from the camaraderie with other breast cancer survivors who may be at different stages in their breast cancer treatment. Healing support can result from the communication that occurs during art therapy if done in a group setting. Art therapists work with many different media, including paper, paint, pencil, crayons, clay, metals, and beads. Not only is it a creative way to express oneself, but it also helps to resolve conflicts and problems by reducing stress and increasing self-awareness. Often art therapy can act as an inner expression of buried emotions through the process of creating. It is a safe way to express emotions that come with breast cancer treatment, and can also help build self-esteem. Art therapy can often be fun and it can be rewarding to see what has been created in the midst of your cancer treatments.

Diet

Diet is not technically a complementary therapy, but more of a foundation for creating a good environment within your body that will promote health and healing and prepare your body for wellness. Diet is about choices that promote health with anti-inflammatory foods and low glycemic foods that lower sugar levels to reduce the levels of IGF (insulin growth factor). Making better choices helps create an environment that is anti-cancer in nature.

Experts believe that a typical anti-cancer diet should consist of fish; organic meat; omega-3 eggs; organic dairy products; multigrain breads; vegetables; fruits; olive, canola, or flaxseed oil; and fresh herbs and spices. Choosing these healthy food alternatives helps create an anti-cancer environment within your body. It is recommended that you eat sugar and white flour sparingly, instead using agave nectar and multigrain flour. Avoid all hydrogenated vegetable fats—trans fats—and all animal fats loaded with omega-6s.

CHAPTER 12

Positive Mental Attitude

Recent studies point to a resurgence in using positive psychology, which focuses on ways to look at your situation with a positive outlook. The studies find that a positive outlook and attitude can be cultivated in your life, even if you are in a negative place. E. P. Seligman, PhD, writes in his book, *Authentic Happiness,* that optimistic people tend to interpret their troubles as transient and controllable, whereas pessimistic people believe that their troubles last forever and are uncontrollable. He explains that optimism is a strength that helps promote well-being. Seligman calls this optimism a mature defense to help in the process of living. This chapter will explore how to develop and cultivate a positive mental attitude while going through your breast cancer journey.

Develop a Positive Mental Attitude

Developing and cultivating a positive mental attitude comes from looking at your world differently and purposefully. Optimism in positive psychology is considered a core virtue. For example, wisdom, knowledge, courage, love, humanity, justice, temperance, spirituality, and transcendence are core values that create optimism. Medicine and psychology examines the body and mind, but often neglect the spiritual realm, which is more difficult to measure.

159

The feeling of well-being that has been discussed with the use of complementary therapies—its effect on the immune system, easing side effects of cancer treatment, and the enhanced feeling—promote a deeper relaxation response. This deep relaxation response is also one of the outcomes of practicing positive psychology. It is a general feeling of life-force energy that promotes health and well-being.

L. Essential

The best way to predict your future is to create it. Creating your own Shangri-La in life is another way to say that you can create and react to the situations in your life with an optimistic stance versus a pessimistic one. Experiencing a life-threatening disease such as breast cancer is a challenging feat to take on without a positive attitude. As an added bonus, the Shangri-La you create in life during your breast cancer journey can be with you for life.

Having a positive attitude does not cure your breast cancer, but can make the journey more bearable for you. Many of us can remember older relatives who lived through the Depression and we look at them as people of strength and courage who became resilient through enduring their circumstances. The reality is that those troubled times are what brought that generation's inner strengths to the forefront. You acquire strength through experiences in life and by adapting and changing to survive.

Good health is considered one of the keys to happiness and well-being. However, cultivating learned optimism is also a key to achieving good health. Consider for example, the pessimistic viewpoint—"Having breast cancer is overwhelming, I can't believe I have breast cancer"—versus an optimistic viewpoint—"I am living with breast cancer right now in my life and I am going to get through it."

Cultivating an attitude of gratitude and hope can be challenging when going through breast cancer treatment. To cultivate means just that—it is a learned and acquired talent that anyone can nurture and grow within themselves. To cultivate optimism and hope is to look at life differently. Review your signature strengths and virtues (those qualities that you know in your heart that you possess). By engaging those qualities in your current situation, you can foster feelings of well-being and strength. Instead of your daily "things to do" list, keep a "gratitude" list. No matter what situation you find yourself in, there are people in your life, strengths and virtues you possess, for which you can exercise the spirit of gratitude.

 Fact

The mind-body connection is well known in the health care arena. The mind influences the body's reaction to illness and its resilience is based on healthy coping strategies, and one's ability to fight off stress, thus building the body's immune system against disease.

Developing strengths and virtues focuses on growth of the inner being and not on those things that are physical and outward, such as one's appearance. Therefore, when loss seems to be the residing theme—loss of your previous life as you know it, loss of your perception of good health, and perhaps the loss of your breasts and the temporary loss of your hair—you can focus on inner growth of your signature strengths and virtues. In reality, our outward physical appearances decline with age and focusing on developing our inner strengths and virtues means that they will only get better with time.

Choose to Find Hope in All You Do

Hope is the concept of looking at your situation in a positive light. It is difficult to measure and, like humor, is very subjective. You must recognize that you can choose to have hope, and that this choice takes as much energy as choosing to see the dark side of life, which lends itself to feeling more helpless.

Hope presents itself when your situation can go either way. When you look at your breast cancer journey in a hopeful way, your perspective about your situation changes. Stephen Jay Gould, a professor at Harvard University who had two incidences of mesothelioma of the abdomen, reported that because he was a scientist, he knew that the statistics were against him and that the median survival rate for his cancer was eight months. He theorized that meant half of the people with the disease lived more than eight months. He then looked at his strengths and good health before his diagnosis and decided that he had every right to believe that he was on the hopeful half of the survival curve. Stephen Jay Gould died from another disease twenty years after his mesothelioma diagnosis. Cancer statistics are guides that do not take into account an individual's unique characteristics and will to live. They also do not show those that just accept the statistics and those who actively reinforce their own natural defenses to help give them a more favorable outcome.

It is important to be aware of the statistics, but also to look at the positive side of the statistics to learn the percentage of recurrence or survival. Statistics help guide the doctor and you to develop your breast cancer treatment plan. Choosing hope and cultivating an optimistic view during your breast cancer journey will make you feel better. This requires an active participation in promoting health, finding meaning to your experience, and inner peace with your life circumstances.

Do Whatever It Takes to Stay Positive

Staying positive—looking at your circumstances in your favor—takes focus, determination, and courage. Increasing optimism and hope is an acquired and learned skill. For some, going about their daily routine with some moderation is best, while for others, exploring complementary therapies and developing new ways to cope and stay healthy during treatments is better. Engaging the mind and body can help you stay in a centered and balanced place in the manner that you enjoy best.

 Alert

Making the choice to train your mind to look at breast cancer as a temporary problem helps to keep you rational and focused during your breast cancer treatments. Learning to argue with yourself when negative thoughts enter your mind and replace them with good thoughts, visualizing a peaceful scene, and using deep breathing techniques or yoga practices, are all strategies that can have lifelong benefits.

To increase optimism, you may have to combat the old negative messages and thoughts that come to mind. For example, "I have nothing good in my life; everything has been going wrong all my life and now I have breast cancer; I am doomed," demonstrates a pessimistic outlook. To increase optimism, try to change your way of thinking, and say to yourself, "Having breast cancer has changed my life and my focus for now. I will get through this part of my life and eventually will have it behind me." It gives breast cancer a temporary place in your life and gives you a more optimistic view. This is a healthier way to look at your breast cancer. Breast cancer does not deserve to be all-encompassing or to define who you are, but should be seen only as a part of your life for now. Having breast cancer can help incorporate new and healthful strategies and wisdom in your life.

Life Is a Process, so Is Having Breast Cancer

Many existential philosophers theorize that all of life's circumstances and experiences add to our perception of and meaning to our lives. Victor Frankl, a psychotherapist and concentration camp survivor, developed logotherapy from his experience and based it on finding one's meaning of life as its philosophy. In his book, *Man's Search for Meaning,* he purports that each of us is "questioned by life," and that each can only find the answer to life by "answering for his own life," and that each one "can only respond by being responsible." Ask yourself what this situation of having breast cancer is asking of you. What are you to learn from this? Has this experience enriched you in any way?

L. Essential

In existential psychology, the anxiety and angst that come with breast cancer should work constructively as a motive for change and growth. Be patient with yourself during this journey. It is life-altering and life-changing and you are in control of its meaning and its purpose for you.

On life's journey, a disability, emotional trauma, breast cancer, or any life-threatening event that compromises our quality of life teaches us what we are destined to learn. You have to determine what life's meaning is to you. Recognizing that you have the power of choice, the gift of self-awareness, and that you are a unique and special person, can bring meaning to life. Abraham Maslow taught about self-actualization as the highest level of being once your basic needs have been met and you have come into yourself. But self-transcendence is of a higher level than self-actualization, in which one looks outside oneself to a higher purpose for being.

Surround Yourself with Positive People

There are always the "downers" in your life: the friends and family members who find the worst-case scenario in every situation, and have chosen a pessimistic view of life. At times, we all have this view of life. However, it's how much we let it invade our minds and take up residence there that matters. You can help keep the negativity at bay by not allowing another person's negative view of the world to influence yours. Conversely, if there are people in your life who lift you up, make it your business to be around them. This will help your frame of mind while you are going through breast cancer treatments and helps put you in a position of strength. Positivity breeds positivity, so surround yourself with a network of positive people and a support team. Try to limit your time with those who have the gloom-and-doom mentality. Practice self-care—you need to think of yourself and make good choices as to the company you keep.

One way to find positive people in your life is to cultivate a positive outlook yourself, which will attract positive people like a magnet. When you are in the midst of your breast cancer treatment, such an attitude can be a challenging goal. You can develop a positive attitude by incorporating the message of positivity in your life. To do this, you can make up your own mantra or use the following, changing it to suit your own situation. Let it be your new mantra and just sit and watch what happens next and who comes into your life.

Living with breast cancer mantra:

- I have decided to live.
- I am done with my preoccupation and obsession with my breast cancer diagnosis.
- I choose hope in all aspects of my life, including my breast cancer journey.
- I want to live joyfully and fruitfully today, tomorrow, and every day.
- I believe that I am bigger than this breast cancer and I will survive.
- I can control the emotional, psychological, and spiritual aspects of having breast cancer.

- I believe that breast cancer is only a part of my life's journey and not all of it.
- I want to teach from my experience and move on to the more resilient, strong, and complete woman that I am to be.
- I believe that having breast cancer is a message for me to change and only I can truly know the way.
- I believe that I can go through the breast cancer journey, its treatment, and its effects on my body, its impact on my mind and spirit and deep within my soul.
- I will vow in my heart to live in peace with myself, the important people in my life and in my world, and with my God.
- I will participate in life and not be on the sidelines as an observer or just going along for the ride.
- I will trust my instincts and my personal power to overcome.
- I will forgive myself for my shortcomings and forgive others.
- I choose to be happy in spite of myself at times.
- I will spend my quality time with positive people and those who are in my circle of support.
- I will remember to not slip back into my old ways prior to having breast cancer. I am a new person! I will season with the gift of time.
- I will remember to schedule quiet time for myself as I journey through my breast cancer treatment and listen to the stillness of the moments in my life.
- I will always be there for those women who follow in my footsteps.

What to Do When You Encounter Negative People in Your Life

You may meet negative people as often as positive ones. It is your choice who you fill your life with. Once you are in a position of strength, you may even be able to teach others about cultivating positivity in their own lives. Negativity is toxic, and as breast cancer survivors, we can identify with toxins. First, you must prepare yourself against them, by keeping your body, mind, and spirit healthy so that you will recognize negativity as it tries to sneak in. You can use some of the techniques you learned during your breast cancer treatments, such as mindful meditation, focusing your breath, prayer, and centering yourself. Visualize a bubble around you so that you can be present with negative forces and yet not let them find a way into your life. Recognize that your life force and energy is comprised of all that is good, natural, and peaceful and you need to protect it.

CHAPTER 13

Opportunities

The questions that each person with breast cancer must ask
herself are: What is the breast cancer experience teaching me?
What is the meaning of my life here on earth and how do I want
to live now and in the future? What is important to me personally?
The breast cancer journey brings self-awareness, growth, and wisdom and can help you live a fuller and more enriched life. This
chapter will look at the opportunities that breast cancer brings.

In All of Life's Crises Lie Opportunities

No one who is first diagnosed with breast cancer can ever imagine
that having breast cancer can bring opportunities. Opportunities
come when you least expect them. They depend on you and usually come when you are ready to receive them. Being open to new
experiences, meeting new people, and getting acquainted in a personal way with the health care world brings new circumstances
and decisions, and helps you decide what is important to you.

You are empowered to do what you choose according to the
opportunities that present themselves. Dealing with breast cancer, which is a life-altering experience, brings many changes and
adjustments. The prospect of having your breasts removed will
never be considered an opportunity unless your breast reconstruction presents you with the breasts you may have had in the past.

Others may see their breast cancer as an opportunity to reduce their breasts. Whatever circumstance you find yourself in during treatment, you have the freedom to evaluate it, address it, and then do as your heart, mind, and spirit direct you.

Evaluate What Is Important to You

Reviewing what you value as important helps to eliminate the unimportant. Evaluating and looking at your life and how you spend your time and money, helps you to identify what is truly important to you. It may be your husband, partner, family, children, or friends with whom you invest most of your time. For some it may be their life's work they may want to redirect. It may include your love of cooking, or golfing, or other favorite pastime. As you assess your life and what you spend your time doing, you may find that these things no longer suit your present needs. The realization that life is temporary may change your career goals and the importance that you previously placed on your work accomplishments and financial net worth and status.

Identifying your new life goals is step one in the process of making changes. Finding the strength to make those changes takes time, focus, and determination. Life after breast cancer treatment evolves and you set the pace. You may find that your previous job or career does not fulfill your needs or it just does not mean the same to you. You may find that your passion and drive has changed since your breast cancer experience. What was important to you prior to having breast cancer may be the same. Or it may be much the same but with changes—whether a career change, marriage, having children, or other major life events. The process of change takes planning and, depending on how you want your life to change, will determine how the change will occur. Your shifting perceptions of what you value may initially create conflict until you incorporate those new areas of change into your life.

You may want to exercise more, develop a daily yoga or meditation practice, take up a new hobby such as hiking or birdwatching, or pursue arts and crafts that allow you to enjoy living in the moment. Hobbies and other interests help you to participate and focus on the activity at hand, which rests your mind and spirit. Having a hobby or relaxing interest adds balance to a hectic life schedule and life's responsibilities.

Essential

Maybe you can pursue a hobby that you have always put aside in your life because of competing tugs at your time and other responsibilities. Many have learned new skills or developed a passion that they have always had, such as playing the piano or taking dance lessons. The possibilities are endless. However, you will have to consider your physical limitations and where you are in your breast cancer treatment during your new pursuits.

Find an Opportunity to Reach Out to Others

"The more you lose yourself in something bigger than yourself, the more energy you will have." This quote from Norman Vincent Peale expresses the nature of giving and the blessings that accompany it. Whether you reach out to someone in your neighborhood who is going through breast cancer treatment by making a meal, or offering someone a ride to the doctor, or just a leisurely ride to distract them from the events of the day, every little bit matters. When you are actively receiving breast cancer treatment, you will probably have limited energy for reaching out to others. However, as you begin your recovery, it can help your own healing process to help others.

Volunteer to Help a Local Breast Cancer Cause

Volunteering to help a local breast cancer cause or group does more than get you together with other women and men living with breast cancer, it also helps you in your own healing process. Scientists and researchers in the mind-body connection arena recognize that looking outside oneself to help others also contributes to self-healing. Some research indicates that cancer patients do better overall with their care when they are actively involved in volunteer work for a cause. The act of volunteering makes a person feel good and gives her energy, which contributes to improved perceptions of health. The camaraderie of being with other breast cancer survivors, family and friends, and those who have lost their loved ones to breast cancer, bonds a group of people. Doing something positive in the midst of breast cancer treatment or recovery brings an inner feeling of peace and strengthens one's spirit of hope. Whether you take part in a breast cancer walk, a fund-raising event that you can participate in—like a wine-tasting or jewelry party where the proceeds benefit breast cancer—or some other event, you will not only be giving to an important cause, but also lightening your spirit. It will be one of those priceless moments in your recovery.

Start Your Own Fundraising Event

If you are so moved, you could even start your own fundraising event to help support the breast center where you received your treatment. In the process of receiving your own breast cancer treatment, you may have identified an area of need; for example, a lack of resource books in the chemotherapy room or a support group for children of breast cancer patients. This is more of a grass-roots effort, and some important things to consider if you are thinking of starting your own fundraising project include:

- Contact your local breast cancer center or hospital with your idea.
- Start small.
- Get people on board who have fundraising and marketing experience.
- Recruit family, friends, breast cancer survivors, and other volunteers who will want to join your cause.
- Form a grass-roots steering committee.
- Write a proposal for what you want to accomplish and how, including a time frame and budget for your project. (Remember, this does not have to be a professional proposal but it will act as your strategy and help you to plan with specific objectives in mind. Also, it will help in soliciting local sponsors when they see that it is well-thought-out and you mean business.)
- Solicit local sponsors for start-up money (remember that support can also be in the form of in-kind support such as agreeing to print and supply brochures for a walk, golf tournament, or other fundraiser you are planning).
- You may want to join forces with a distributor of a product line, such as food products or jewelry, and give your percentage of the profits as well as the company's to your breast cancer initiative.

Fundraising for an Established Charity

There are many fun ways to give back to others and organizations who have supported you during your breast cancer treatment. Some ideas to consider are:

- Throw a pasta party and charge admission. You can just ask for a donation without a set price and you will be surprised at your friends' and family's generosity.
- Inquire if your local theater group will donate a percentage of admission to your breast cancer cause and get all your

friends and family involved to attend and help spread the word to others.

- Get your club to do a fundraising event: If you are a biker, do a motorcycle ride for the cure and solicit sponsors, or if you belong to a knitting club or jewelry-making group sell your wares at a local store willing to display your product.

There are so many ways in which you can help make the road a little easier for other women with breast cancer and their families. Recognize that everyone is different and you should only volunteer when you feel emotionally ready and/or you are at a point in your breast cancer journey that you want to reach out to others and take that risk.

 Fact

If there is no local effort that you would like to volunteer for, you can join one of the many national organizations that exist in support of breast cancer causes. For a complete list you can go to: *http:// dir.yahoo.com/Health/Diseases_and_Conditions/Breast_Cancer/ Organizations.*

National Organizations

National organizations tend to be bigger and reach out across geographical areas. For example the Susan G. Komen Breast Cancer Foundation, which started locally, now has many locations that do fundraisers for breast cancer research. Their major fundraiser is a road race called "Race for the Cure."

Another big fundraiser is the two-day Avon Walk. It is more time-intensive and requires that a walker raise money to be eligible to participate. The Avon Foundation provides grants to local, regional, and national breast cancer organizations to support five key areas: awareness and education, screening and diagnosis;

access to support services, and scientific research. The American Cancer Society also has a breast cancer walk in many areas called "Making Strides against Breast Cancer."

It is important to research the organization that you would like to join to make sure that you agree with its mission and what the money is targeted for. There are special interest organizations that may interest you, such as the Young Survival Coalition, which involves a group of survivors that focus on the issues that young women with breast cancer encounter. Some organizations focus on environmental issues and support research and education of the effect of environmental factors on breast cancer.

A good place to start is to find out what is being done in your area, take into account your personal interests and passion, and get involved.

Breast Cancer Awareness and the Pink Ribbon

Once you or someone you love has been diagnosed with breast cancer, everything seems to be coming up pink as you become immersed in the world of breast cancer awareness. Is the color simply a media blitz or does it symbolize what it was intended to do; that is, to create a way to provide both financial and personal support to those who have breast cancer? How did the pink ribbon come to symbolize breast cancer awareness?

The ribbon is a symbol used to connote awareness and support. It had its origins in the yellow ribbon used in the early to mid-1900s in a United States military marching song. Then the song "Tie a Yellow Ribbon" inspired Penney Laingen, the wife of one of the hostages held in Iran from 1979–1981, to use the yellow ribbon to show support for her husband and other hostages and to remind others of their plight. Her family and friends joined her in her efforts and today Americans continue to use this symbol as a powerful reminder of the men and women who are serving our country abroad.

In the past decade or so, many different colored ribbons have become the medium for bringing about awareness. For example, AIDS activists use the red ribbon to show their support. During the Oscar and Tony awards ceremonies, which recognize achievement in American entertainment, many of the celebrities in attendance have donned red ribbons to bring awareness and support of this important cause to a wide audience.

 Fact

The first color to represent breast cancer awareness was not pink, but peach. Peach ribbons were distributed by Charlotte Hayley, who provided them along with a card inviting women to join together to make a statement to politicians in particular, and to Americans in general, that more dollars were needed for breast cancer prevention.

The cosmetics industry got on board in 1991 to promote breast cancer awareness with the help of Evelyn Lauder of Estée Lauder Cosmetics and Alexander Penney, the editor-in-chief of *SELF* magazine. When Evelyn Lauder and Alexander Penney were working on their breast cancer awareness promotion, they liked Charlotte Hayley's concept of giving ribbons to promote the support of breast cancer awareness. Lauder, Penney, and Hayley worked together to come up with the pink ribbon symbol for breast cancer awareness.

The first breast cancer organization to hand out pink ribbons was the Susan G. Komen Race for the Cure, which handed out the ribbons to runners at its annual road race in the fall of 1991 in New York City.

Today, the pink ribbon is synonymous with the breast cancer effort and continues to serve as a symbol of awareness, education, and support, not only during October, which is Breast

Cancer Awareness Month, but throughout the year. Marketing has taken this concept to such a high level that one may begin to dislike the color because of the commercialization of the cause. The market is inundated with pink products used in breast cancer fundraising efforts. From the traditional clothing items such as T-shirts, hats, socks, and jackets to pink dice, playing cards, jewelry, and golf balls, to food products such as gummy ribbons, M&Ms, pink cocktail drinks—the list goes on. Even the United States Postal Service has a breast cancer stamp that supports the cause. For anyone who has gone through breast cancer treatments, pink has its purpose. Many feel that wearing pink may trigger someone's memory to get a mammogram, to raise awareness of the disease, show that it is an important cause to many men and women, and to raise money for patient support and for research for its cure.

 In Her Own Words

I have developed a strong dislike for the color pink. Especially pink ribbons. Being a "girlie girl," I always thought pink was a pretty color. But, immediately after my diagnosis, I saw pink ribbons were everywhere. I found myself becoming offended at the sight of pink ribbons on cars because on the rare occasions during treatment when I wasn't thinking about cancer (or my next infusion, or a doctor appointment, or a test result, etc.), I would see a pink ribbon on the back of someone's car and BOOM! There it was—right in my face.

—Chelsey, age 41, 2-year survivor

There are also anti–pink breast cancer advocacy groups, such as Breast Cancer Action in San Francisco, which encourages people to "do something besides shop," and emphasizes that the amount of money spent on theme advertising would be better spent going directly to research. The group also sports buttons that are black and red and say "Cancer Sucks," delivering a much more direct message and certainly an ice-breaker in conversations about breast cancer. The group also focuses on environmental factors that might contribute to breast cancer, such as toxins used in the cosmetic industry and other commercial applications that promote cancer's growth, delivering the message that prevention of breast cancer needs to be the goal. Some proponents of the anti–pink ribbon concept feel that the color pink connotes a soft and feminine image and that the fight against breast cancer requires a bold, aggressive message to make an impact on this disease.

In general, one should always look at where the money goes for the pink promotional items you buy and what percentage goes to breast cancer support, research, etc. Also examine the integrity of the companies that you support to determine if they are environmentally friendly in their methods.

Essential

Did you know you can buy a pink and white striped mattress made by Vera Wang and that there is a Delta pink plane to support breast cancer? From bed to plane, you can quietly lay your body down at night on it or you can fly in the pinkness of breast cancer awareness. But the choice is always yours!

Whether you go with the pink flow or not will depend on your personality and where you are in your breast cancer treatment. Recognizing that there are as many different ways to support breast cancer awareness as there are different ways to reach people from various backgrounds, the important end result of raising awareness and increasing support is to find a cure for breast cancer and, better yet, prevent its occurrence.

Discover the Wisdom That Cancer Brings

Having breast cancer or any life-threatening disease leads to a journey of discovery of the unknown experiences that produce change, adaptation, and growth. As you incorporate these experiences into your being, you develop a wisdom that is uniquely yours. The journey of self-awareness, facing your fears, coping with difficulties, and learning to live in the face of adversity brings wisdom. Wisdom that comes from the cancer experience can be shared by writing a memoir, or journal, which has been proven to decrease anxiety, and provides a self-healing process to the breast cancer journey. If you found journaling to be helpful, you might volunteer to be a guest speaker at a breast cancer support group and do a journaling workshop geared toward breast cancer issues and concerns.

You may want to become a mentor for someone who is at the beginning stages of her breast cancer treatment. You might make yourself available to answer any questions she may have or at least refer her to someone who can help. You can volunteer at your local breast center by letting your health care professionals know that you are willing to help. Check with your breast cancer center. They may need volunteers to hold someone's hand during breast biopsies, or have ideas for many other ways you can help make the journey easier for others.

Living Life the Way It Was Meant to Be Lived

Human nature for many reasons focuses on living. People are busy making plans, setting financial goals, establishing career moves, building a family life, and not dwelling on the end. Often much time is wasted on unimportant things that are valued at that moment or time in your life. Having breast cancer brings your mortality to the forefront. What your beliefs have been before now may be questioned as the reality sets in that our life on earth is only temporary.

Life is meant to be lived. You are a unique partner in life with purpose and meaning to your existence, so why not live it with a participatory viewpoint? It is easier to prioritize the important things, experiences, and people in your life when you have dealt firsthand with breast cancer. You can choose to waste less time or waste more time. Spend less time at work and more time enjoying your family and friends. You may decide to finally go on that trip you have been putting off for so long.

L, Essential

Living with the end in mind is one way to participate in your life with a zest, awareness, and appreciation that may go unnoticed prior to having breast cancer. Being diagnosed with breast cancer is not a gift in itself, but the wisdom that comes from the experience is a gift that can enrich and fulfill your life. Life is meant to be lived with the thought that "life is not a dress rehearsal—you only have one chance at it."

Once you have come face to face with your mortality, then you can truly live. In that spirit, Debbie Mazza-Taylor, who lost her five-year battle with breast cancer just days before her forty-first birthday, wrote this poem:

> For what is it to die but to stand naked in the wind?
> And to melt into the sun
> And what is it to cease breathing, but to free the breath
> From its restless tides, that it may rise and expand
> Seeking God unencumbered?
> Only when you drink from the river of silence
> Shall you indeed sing.
> And when you have reached the mountaintop
> Then you shall begin to climb.
> And when earth shall claim your limbs,
> Then shall you truly dance.

CHAPTER 14

Empowerment and Capturing Your "New Normal"

Feeling empowered is subjective and varies from individual to individual. But the universal truth of empowerment comes from the knowledge that you have options and control over your choices; the ability to make those choices, and the responsibility for the choices you make. Empowerment is that feeling and conviction that comes from having gone through a difficult situation and made it. Capturing your "new normal" is taking that newly empowered self and using it to form a new and improved you. The way you viewed yourself in the world and how you filled your days prior to having breast cancer will take on new meaning. Your perspective may not change at all, but for most women living with breast cancer, the experience enriches their lives and takes life down a new path. This chapter is about finding empowerment no matter what stage of breast cancer treatment you are in and then using it to create a "new normal" for yourself.

Your Greatest Growth Comes from Your Greatest Difficulties

One of the greatest difficulties in life is facing one's own mortality. Living with breast cancer and the uncertainty of its outcome can be a time of emotional, physical, and spiritual upheaval in one's life. It is often said that with great difficulties comes personal growth. This personal growth and strength can also bring a sense of accomplishment: "I made it, I finished my chemotherapy and radiation treatments and I am here to talk about it." You reflect on what you have learned. The breast cancer experience brings you to another place that you don't encounter in normal everyday life. It is an experience that stands alone and is set apart from everything else that has ever happened to you.

Often others will say how much they admire you for the strength you showed in coping with breast cancer. Accept and be proud of not only getting through breast cancer treatments but also for the wisdom the experience has taught you. You are now in a position to give back and it will feel good. You can choose to empower others, share what worked for you during your breast cancer treatment, and offer encouragement to someone who has been newly diagnosed. Empowerment knows that no matter what situation you are in that there is always something positive you can do.

No one chooses to grow by facing life's difficulties, but this is how empowerment begins and together with personal growth you emerge as a person with courage, empowered to be your true self.

Essential

"In the long run, we shape our lives, and we shape ourselves. The process never ends until we die. And the choices we make are ultimately our own responsibility." —Eleanor Roosevelt

The Many Faces of Breast Cancer

Empowering yourself is a learned art and not a science. It is an empirical openness that usually comes from the deep struggles within you. There are many books available to teach the tools of empowerment and you are encouraged to embark on that journey. It can be as simple or complex as you choose it to be. You may find a whole new world of spirituality and a ministry to share with others or you may be a source of strength and knowledge for those who follow in your path.

The struggles and difficulties that the diagnosis of breast cancer brings take on many faces and add facets to your life that lead to the empowering spirit within you:

- The warrior face that initially begins the battle within you
- The reflective face that begins when you turn inward and look back at the past experiences in your life to try to make sense of it all
- The face of the unknown of what lies ahead
- The face of being lied to about being a victim of breast cancer
- The face of an all-knowing and peaceful being that has seasoned along with your breast cancer
- The face of survivorship, a bond you have with other cancer survivors
- The face of empowerment that gives hope to yourself and others

Here are ten ways to empower yourself:

1. Take responsibility.
2. Focus on the difficulty at hand and don't submit to the "all or nothing" theory.
3. Be optimistic.
4. Look for creative solutions.
5. Have courage.
6. Take heart—remember empowerment lies from within.
7. Take action.
8. Determine that you can overcome.
9. Think ahead—know that this too will pass.
10. Be open to what lies ahead.

Overcoming Your Fears

In the process of empowering oneself, overcoming your fears becomes paramount. Fears foster a polarity in your mind—they are at odds with the empowering spirit within. Fear involves the memory or thought of what is feared and the emotional attachment associated with that fear. Breast cancer recurrence is one of the major fears that plague women who have had breast cancer. One technique to use is that when fear arises, you need to neutralize it in order to help dissipate its emotional hold. It is the same concept that employers teach about dealing with angry and difficult customers. You need to dissipate their anger with a calm approach. First you acknowledge their frustration, listen, and then jointly come to a resolution by verifying the results of your actions with the customer. In the same way, you are working to dissipate your fears by acknowledging them, listening, and then coming to terms with your fears by taking action.

 Fact

> Whether it is the fear of recurrence, passing a gene along to your daughter, or fear of your own mortality and the unknown, you can empower yourself to conquer the fear and fill yourself with good energy from the positive people in your life, the nature around you, or engaging in energy work such as Reiki, yoga, Pilates, meditation, and prayer.

A simple technique to help combat the fears that you may have regarding your breast cancer is to take your fear and visualize it as being put it onto a stone or an object. Then acknowledge the fear, accept it, sit with it, and then throw it away visually or physically. You will find this a freeing experience and you may need to gently remind yourself that it is gone. You can even have a going-away party for it. You can invite your friends or party alone, the choice is up to you—the empowered you.

Find Out What Is Important to You

As discussed in the previous chapter, you have identified your priorities and have made the necessary changes that you wanted and now those relationships, things, and opportunities that you value become your focus. Living by enjoying those things, people, and treasured memories brings clear direction and clarification to your everyday life. Writing down what is most important to you, not just thinking about it, will bring clarity to what you feel is important. This is what is called purposeful living, or having a value-driven life. This process involves self-reflection by identifying what is important to you. Purpose flows from values that are shaped by your past, your upbringing, your parents' influence, and your environment and circumstances in life. Whenever a decision is made, whether consciously or unconsciously, these values affect all you do.

There is no judgment made once you have assessed what you find important to you. It may be your job, a pet, family, friends, or a favorite pastime that motivates you to spend more time doing what you enjoy. Your list may look something like this:

- Family
- Financial security
- Career
- Happiness
- Love
- A summer home to retire to
- Traveling

Once you have made your personal list, you may want to share it with your partner, spouse, and children. You may even want to change your priority list based on what you have discovered from those closest to you. After all, they will be the ones who will share in the joys as well as the challenges in your life.

One way to find out what is important to you is to look at what you spend your time doing and spend your money on. This will give you clues to what you value. If you don't like what you see—i.e., you spend too much time at work or watch too much TV—you may want to take another look at this and make some life changes. It is all up to you. Remember, no judgments are allowed: Only be true to yourself and recognize that the choices you make are shaped by what you value. There are no good or bad choices, only better ones to achieve your personal goals.

 Alert

Financial planners know the secrets of goal planning—knowing what you want to achieve, strategizing, and reassessing your plan. Finding out what is important to you is a road map to life planning. It can provide a clear direction and path to your life.

Prioritize Your Needs

The next step is to review the things you have identified as important and prioritize them by levels of importance. By numbering or categorizing them, you will be able to internalize what you have written into your daily life. For example, if your family is the most important priority, then spend quality time with them during and after your breast cancer treatments. If you have always wanted to travel and can afford it, go ahead and do it with the people you want to be with most.

Know You Are in the Driver's Seat

Think about this—no one can really make the decision about your breast cancer treatments. The decision lies with you. Your friends and family will have their own ideas about what is best for you but only you can determine the path you take. You alone are responsible for the choices that you are most comfortable with and are able to live with. There is no one right road to take, perhaps just a better one for you. Once you realize this concept, whether you change the route or go somewhere you hadn't planned—you are still driving the bus. Recognize and believe this to be true. Set the stage for feeling empowered throughout your breast cancer journey. The people on your bus have bought tickets and you have chosen the ones who are to ride along with you. They may change seats or positions in your life during the journey, some may even get off or on at various stops and others remain for the duration through it all. The important thing to remember is that you are driving the bus. Your physical, psychological, and emotional needs as well as your attitude, all determine the kind of ride you will experience.

When You Feel Like Someone Else Is Driving

The people in your circle of support are powerful influences in your life and may think they know exactly what you should do or better yet, what they would do if they were in your situation. This is when you may need to put a stop to those messages and get back into the driver's seat. Many are well-intentioned, so being kind in your responses is always the better way to go. If you are someone who normally likes to be driven around and are more comfortable when others take charge, well, this is the time in your life that is worth the effort to make all of your own decisions, especially when the doctor is talking about your life. This is your life and you only have one chance to live it. People who you respect may want to guide you by their own sets of values and priorities. They may have your best interest at heart but only *you* know what is best for you. Taking responsibility for being the driver is probably the most difficult aspect of your breast cancer journey.

How to Make Yourself the Driver Again

Listening to your loved ones' advice helps to get your engine running, especially those whom you have respected and who have been part of your everyday life. Seeking advice and counsel from these special people is always a good start in forming your own plan of action and gives you food for thought. However, it is important to remember that each individual forms his or her decisions based on their own life experiences, so you need to take this into account once you have sought the opinions of others about what is best for you. Making yourself the driver again takes courage and is hard work and requires energy at a time in your life when your energy level is being challenged by breast cancer treatments, work, and your personal life. Listen to your inner compass. This is the core of your heart's work, which brings a sense of peace when you make yourself the driver again.

Listen to Your Heart and Follow It

While being treated for breast cancer, you may be focused on the medical and scientific aspects of the disease and neglect the heart of the matter. The intuition of the heart and spirit can lead you to a place of inner peace. Honing in on what your heart is telling you is a learned talent that develops from your unique life force. The oneness you have of heart, mind, body, and spirit comes from inner work and centering practices. Your heart dictates your gut feelings about what is happening in and to your body. Listening to the cues, whether it is to relax, to spend time with a friend who brings you comfort, or getting a massage, all help you to be in tune with what your body is telling you. If you are fatigued and have no energy to keep going, that is when you need to relax, sit down, and restructure your priorities. Our body has the capacity to heal itself. It lets you know when something is wrong. Being in tune with your body's needs during breast cancer treatments will help you adjust and transition to listening to your body and responding in a healthful way.

In His Own Words

When my aunt (who is only a few years old than me) was diagnosed, I quickly figured out that being supportive meant my saying less and listening more . . . showing up, being present, helping her figure it out. And when she was ready, I coached her to move beyond the science.

—Michael, nephew of Lucy, 16-year survivor

Only you know where you want to go and who you want to bring with you on the ride. Once you are empowered, you are free to go where you wish. It is a journey that values all of life's experiences, including having breast cancer. Having breast cancer is only one aspect of your life's journey that makes your journey uniquely yours. No one but you has experienced the same past, environment, social conditions, joys, and struggles, so therefore it is your ride to live. The empowerment that emerges when you have lived through breast cancer treatment is knowing that you have faced your mortality and have lived, and that you will live each day with appreciation.

The Benefits of Living Your Life with Purpose and Design

Knowing what is important to you and living by your values helps to reduce stress that comes from the conflicting values of believing and wanting one thing and living another. You need to reflect on the three major areas where you spend your resources:

1. Your schedule
2. Your budget
3. Your relationships

Once you reflect on those three areas, eliminate the things that don't matter. Stop doing what isn't important to you so that you will have time, money, and energy to do the things that are most important to you. This is the benefit of living your life with purpose and design. Other benefits of this lifestyle are that it helps you to make decisions in your life, gives you a sense of purpose and direction, creates focus, and attracts other people to your life that complement your purpose. Knowing what is important to you and defining your purpose prepares you to take an inventory of where you are in the process of working toward that purpose.

Accept That Your Old Self Is No Longer

The thing that many women have in common after breast cancer treatment is a sense that they don't feel the same as they did before breast cancer. The effects of surgical and medical treatment may continue for some time. Routine follow-up appointments usually continue for up to five years after diagnosis and treatment. Having learned about common concerns and knowing the physical changes that your body has been through, it is unlikely that you will feel the same as you did before your breast cancer diagnosis. You can feel healthy again: It's just going to take much longer than you might anticipate, usually six months to a year after treatment. You may have lost one or both of your breasts; you may have had lymph node surgery, chemotherapy, radiation, or both. You may have had breast reconstructive surgery and your body image has changed during your breast cancer treatment plan. Your definition of feeling healthy most likely has changed after undergoing breast cancer treatment. With all this in mind it is normal to not feel your old self.

After breast cancer treatment you may experience your hair growing back and your body may be thrust into early menopause at an accelerated rate as a result of chemotherapy. These contributing factors change your definition of what is "normal" for you. Two of the common aftereffects of breast cancer treatment are difficulty with focus and memory "chemobrain," and fatigue that seems to linger long after your last chemotherapy or radiation treatment.

 Fact

Everyone is different, but you can expect a recovery period to be at least as long as your breast cancer treatment. You may not feel exactly as you did pre–breast cancer. You can expect a new feeling of health and normalcy that is different, but not necessarily worse. As you begin your life after breast cancer, you should have a sense of your new energy level and begin to feel more comfortable with the process back to your "new normal."

The learned coping strategies that you developed during breast cancer treatment can help you cope with those after-cancer changes that stick around perhaps for a lifetime. The fear of recurrence that lingers on long after breast cancer treatment as well as becoming menopausal as a result of chemotherapy requires acceptance and adaptation. Managing your expectations can help to decrease the stress associated with these changes.

Identifying What Your "New Normal" Is

Even though family, friends, and coworkers may want you to get back to your old self by resuming your previous activities, the process of identifying what your "new normal" is will take time. It is a good idea to make sure that those around you understand that just because your breast cancer treatments are over doesn't mean that you can just jump back into your previous activities and workload; resuming your eight-to ten- hour work day, carpooling, coaching games, etc. In fact, you may discover that in this stage after breast cancer treatment that you can only comfortably do one extracurricular activity a week in addition to your day-to-day responsibilities.

This stage of recuperation after breast cancer treatment is your chance to restructure your life and make choices that will have an impact on how you live the rest of your life. You may decide to slow down your pace, perhaps not work so hard, or spend more time with family and friends. Another important fact is that most breast cancer survivors are sensitive to what their body is telling them and every ache and pain may bring cause for concern. The feeling that your body failed you before promotes this hypersensitivity to anything that feels foreign to you.

After breast cancer treatment your body feels different, especially if you have had reconstructive surgery, chemotherapy, or radiation. Also, chemo-induced menopause will most surely make you feel differently. Your hormonal makeup, if you have had anti-estrogen therapy, will contribute to a foreign or "new normal" feeling of well-being. Identifying your "new normal" takes time and patience and is a long process that begins after your breast cancer treatments are over.

Deciding How You Want to Live the Rest of Your Life

This life-altering experience of having breast cancer cannot be ignored and life just does not go on as it did before you had breast cancer. It is a time when you have to get back that trust you had in your body prior to having breast cancer.

Going forward, you begin to examine how you live your life and question all you do. You may decide that you want to make changes. You may decide that you are going to learn how to say no to many of the activities that previously consumed your time and zapped your energy.

The breast cancer journey is a struggle as well as a gift. The insight you gain from the experience can help you begin a new journey of the new you, valuing and making the most of each day.

Breast Cancer as a Motivator for Change

Once you have coped with cancer, your life is never the same. Because of the life-altering nature of breast cancer, many women tell about the minor and major changes that their cancer has inspired. Some women may find themselves taking on a new career, or looking at their family relationships and perhaps changing them if they find them to be toxic in their life. Other cancer survivors find themselves pursuing new leisure activities as well as other interests and hobbies. Cancer changes the way you look at your life and you most likely had never thought so much about your limited time on earth until your breast cancer diagnosis. You may find yourself acutely aware of how finite life is and feel propelled to make changes in your life. Your breast cancer has made you realize how much time you have wasted lamenting over past hurts and losses. Now you want to make the best use of your time and the pendulum seems to swing dramatically in the other direction.

 In Her Own Words

I was diagnosed in November 1999. Two surgeries and endless weeks of radiation left me so badly burned and exhausted, I thought I would never survive. I will be forever grateful to my husband, friends, and all the brave women I met through a local breast cancer support program. Not a day goes by that I don't give thanks for still being here and being healthy.

—Kathi, age 54, 9-year survivor

Your view of things has changed and you become easily frustrated with the insignificant and unimportant aspects of your previous daily routines now that you are on the road of recovery. Breast cancer forces you to not have the same confidence in your body as you did prior to having breast cancer. Many women decide to shift their career to one that is more meaningful and provides them with a better quality of life. You may feel that you are not fulfilled at work, or because of your changing priorities, you embark on furthering your education, changing jobs, or taking on a job with less stress and even less money if necessary. You may even choose different friends or perhaps decide to end a long-term relationship as a result of the changes that have occurred in you. Your relationships often take on new meaning and what met your needs prior to having breast cancer may no longer work for you.

Having breast cancer does come with some barriers that need to be thought through prior to making any major change, especially in your career. You may need to make short-term goals as well as long-term goals when making changes. For example, paying off any medical bills or getting access to health insurance if you want to be self-employed may be challenging when you are making major changes. Slowly providing for these anticipated changes will help you to make your plans accordingly. It is normal to want to move forward quickly and you may feel an overwhelming sense of urgency in your life after breast cancer but it is important to move slowly and strategically when making major changes.

If you are like many breast cancer survivors, your illness has motivated you to change your life both in small and big ways on the job and in your personal life. Some tips to ease into life changes after breast cancer are:

CAREER CHANGES:
- Identify the change that you envision for yourself.
- Examine the reasons and motivation for your change.
- Seek out people's advice that you respect.
- Make short- and long-term goals to achieve your changes.
- Research the career or business that you are pursuing.
- Follow or shadow someone in the career that you are exploring.
- Make an appointment with a career counselor for advice.

- Evaluate what impact the change will have on your life; i.e., insurance coverage, retirement benefits, etc.
- Be realistic in your pursuits, recognizing the value of time and energy that will be needed to achieve your change.
- Evaluate and reflect if this life change is worth it to you.

PERSONAL RELATIONSHIP CHANGES:
- Identify how you want your relationships to change and with whom.
- Examine the reasons and motivation for the change.
- Play out the relationship change in your mind and the consequences it may bring.
- Seek counseling prior to making any drastic changes such as within your marriage or when ending a long-standing relationship in your life.
- Evaluate and reflect if this change in your relationship is worth it to you.

Be Sensitive to Family and Friends as They Adjust

As you try to define your "new normal," family and friends will be looking for the business-as-usual side of you that existed before you had breast cancer—and so will you. You will soon realize that there is really no going back to the way things were before the life-changing experience that you have just survived. The changes in you may seem foreign to your family, friends, and coworkers. Some may appreciate the new you with a different set of priorities, but others would like you to return to your previous life. After all, that is what others are comfortable with and it will take time for them to see you in a different light.

It is not uncommon for others to want things back to their normal state for you because that is the expectation that you helped create. During this post–breast cancer treatment period, being aware of changes in your own priorities and values will help you to be sensitive to others adapting to those changes. You might have been a people-pleaser before your breast cancer diagnosis and now you have a newfound confidence that has evolved from your experience. You may no longer have the need to say yes when asked to volunteer or to do all the extra things that you did previously to win the hearts of others—you no longer find the need to be a super woman. After all, you have just been through breast cancer treatment. Your family and friends may be saying "Okay, that's enough," or "Who are you and what did you do with the old you?" The changes that occur immediately after your breast cancer treatments will feel strong at first but with time you may find yourself converting back to your old self prior to breast cancer. Perhaps a good indication that you have slipped back into your former self is that you find yourself losing that sense of peace you had when you took better care of yourself.

Embracing the Freedom You Deserve

Re-creating your "new normal" is your rite of passage after breast cancer treatment. The experience can free you to live a more enriched and full life. Examining your priorities by writing them down, and choosing your new-and-improved-you, takes courage.

You may no longer have the need to be a people-pleaser or have a hard time saying no to things and activities that take you away from your new priorities, whatever they may be. The freedom to live the way you choose is an exhilarating and well-deserved side effect of breast cancer treatments. You may have always been the one to host holiday parties and now you can be the one who becomes the invited guest at the next holiday celebration.

Breast cancer treatment forces you to conserve your energy, which is a useful post–breast cancer treatment life skill that can help your quality of life as you move forward to a healthy state of body, mind, and spirit.

CHAPTER 15

The Future of Living with Breast Cancer

You may have redefined your priorities or at least know in your heart what is important to you. With your priorities established, you have assessed, identified, and reassessed the changes that are important to you. This chapter will discuss your future and how you get down to the business of life after your breast cancer. The business of life is simply living your life to the fullest with the end in mind. It may sadden you to think of getting your affairs in order, but it will bring peace of mind to you as well as to your loved ones. This chapter will help you look at your future of living with breast cancer in practical as well as fun-loving ways.

Getting Down to the Business of Life

Resuming your routine not only at work but within the family unit may seem foreign to you since your life for the past six months to a year has been filled with your breast cancer treatment. It has consumed your life and feels like it has been your full-time job. It is not uncommon to feel removed from the day-to-day lifestyle that you had before your breast cancer diagnosis.

Making the transition back to work is often a struggle for many reasons. Your energy level is not the same. Your body image may be altered, and your perception of feeling healthy has been severely challenged. There are quality-of-life studies being done to look at problems associated with work re-entry after breast cancer treatments. Work is often associated with feeling "normal" again so it is natural to be anxious to return to your work routine. Most people say they are anxious about how their return to work will play out. Research on work re-entry after breast cancer treatments has found that initially, many find it difficult to cope and concentrate, concerned about their effectiveness at work. It has also been found that the more stressful the job the harder the re-entry can be. The larger the company the more accommodations may be available but a smaller company might be more flexible, depending on your job responsibilities. Fatigue after breast cancer treatment is a common problem that can affect your job performance. Also, physical problems that have resulted from breast cancer treatment such as lymphedema, and frequent follow-up appointments place added stress on both employees and employers and can interfere with workflow.

Going Back to Work

Going back to work and the transition you and your coworkers must make can be difficult for everyone, even casual business and personal acquaintances. You may sense an awkwardness from them and find that they do not know what to say or how to act around you.

 Alert

You can choose what you want to say and how much you want to share. Remember that the job is the same, but you are not. You may feel differently about your work life and have difficulty with it after breast cancer. Making value changes will affect those whom you work with and it may take time for them to adjust to the new and improved you.

It is important to realize that you set the tone for how you want people to react. This is the basic principle to remember to get through this initial phase with grace and minimal stress. If you do not want to talk about the experience, then you set the tone. You can tell someone you trust to let others know this and to spread the word. Or you can prepare an answer for those who may ask how you are feeling and even practice your response before going back to work, if you find yourself getting anxious. Let your response be your new mantra at work or whenever you need to use it. One standard response is to say, "I am fine, and thank you." If you want to talk about your experience then here is your chance. Some find the work environment a safe haven to express their feelings because at home they may be concerned about upsetting their family members.

Essential

The Americans with Disabilities Act (ADA) applies to employers with fifteen or more workers. It prohibits discrimination of anyone with a disability, or history of a disability, and cancer is considered a disability. Before a job offer, an employer cannot ask for a medical exam but only after an offer has been made. The ADA also requires covered employers to make reasonable accommodations for your medical issues.

Humor is always a good start in helping others feel comfortable with your breast cancer. Humor puts others at ease and decreases any anxiety that may be present when you first return to work. Some women may want to publicly thank everyone for their support to create an atmosphere of open communication, put out on the table what others may be thinking, and reassure them that all is well and now you are back. Whatever works for you will work for them as you set the stage.

If you have lost your job because of your illness or were not gainfully employed prior to your diagnosis, finding a new job after breast cancer treatment may be more challenging. It is important for you to know about employment laws in relation to your situation.

Communicating with your employer about your specific needs is critical and you need to be specific about what you need. You should check in regularly with your boss either bi-weekly or monthly to let him know how you are progressing. If you have been terminated unfairly, then you may want to seek the advice of an employment law expert. You can find more information about how the Americans with Disabilities Act (ADA) helps cancer survivors get back to work at the government website, *www.ada.gov.*

Try to conserve your energy during nonworking hours so that you can optimize your energy level while at work. Consider hiring or assigning someone to help with your daily housecleaning, laundry, bill paying, etc., during your transitioning back to work in order to conserve your energy.

What about My 401(k)?

Once you have had a life-altering disease such as breast cancer, what you took for granted—for example—saving for your retirement, is now in question. Do you continue to save for retirement? This is a question that only you can answer. You can consult with your doctor, family, and financial investor on your personal options. Your breast cancer prognosis may or may not influence your decisions. You may decide to continue saving for your spouse, partner, or children, regardless of your prognosis. Your individual situation and goals will guide you with this decision. You may decide that while you are actively undergoing cancer treatment and receiving disability benefits from work at a reduced rate from your normal income that you will not invest in retirement until you are feeling better and go back to work full time. Your human resources department can assist you in these matters.

Continue to Question How You Spend Your Time and Money

After breast cancer treatment there is a healthy questioning of how you previously spent your time and money. You may not place the same value on material possessions like your home, car, and clothing when you feel that your health is at risk. You may find yourself spending less on discretionary items and more on the necessities of life. After breast cancer treatment you may find more time to relax because you value your time more and don't want to waste it. It is healthy to question everything you do and why, as long as it helps you to sort out what is important to you as it will give clarity to your choices. A decision to either get a new car or take a trip will be determined by what is now important to you, according to how your values may be shifted. Before you had breast cancer, the car might seem more important, but now, after cancer, traveling with the people you care about may override buying a car. Often, people put off the very things that will bring enjoyment in life, but once they survive a life-threatening illness, it becomes important to make those choices.

Questioning and evaluating how you spend your time and your money helps you to stay focused in all your activities, both personally and professionally. You take nothing for granted, every possession you have and time given to you is a gift that is to be cherished. You wonder how other people go through life not knowing what you know—the preciousness of life and the gift of yourself that can be given to others.

Reassess the Status of Your Will/HCP/DPOA

If you have had a will prepared by an attorney, you may want to look at it more closely. A will primarily addresses where or to whom you wish your assets to go after your death. A living will, on the other hand, helps you and your loved ones by expressing your end-of-life wishes so that if you are incapacitated, your family and loved ones will carry on your wishes in concert with your doctor.

A health-care proxy (HCP) form can be filled out without the help of an attorney and can be completed at most doctors' offices, hospitals, and health care facilities. An HCP designates another person or persons to act on your behalf in regards to your health care decisions. The person named in your HCP should be someone that you trust to carry out your health care wishes when you cannot. If you appointed a HCP prior to your breast cancer diagnosis and you found that person was ill-equipped to assist you or lacked the knowledge and emotional stamina needed, then you may want to appoint another HCP in the future.

A durable power of attorney (DPOA) is a legal document that can only be prepared by an attorney. The document enables an individual to designate another person, called the attorney-in-fact, to act on his or her behalf, even in the event the individual becomes disabled or incapacitated. In essence, the individual so named is designated to be your financial representative, usually paying your bills and managing your overall fiscal affairs when you are not able because of illness or other health care issues.

If you do not have any of these documents, it is advised that you meet with an attorney to prepare them. If you have done them prior to breast cancer treatment, now is a good time to reassess your wishes. After breast cancer treatment, they will have more meaning and require more detailed attention as you have faced your mortality through your breast cancer journey. They will have more significance to you. By embracing your mortality, you will live more freely and purposefully.

Assess Any Special Considerations and Plan for Them

If you have young children, you may want to consider setting up a living trust. You may also want to set up child-care provisions and decide who will be the guardian of your children if you are a single parent or if both you and your spouse were to pass away. If you have a disabled child or elderly parents that you are caring for, then you may want to make special provisions for them and perhaps start an application for Social Security benefits or other federal or state aid for your loved ones.

It is impossible to plan for every eventuality, but there are always unique situations that you can begin planning for. It will give you peace of mind to know that you have done those things that will result in a positive outcome.

Regardless of the size of your estate, you should consult an estate planning attorney.

 Question

What is my estate?
An estate is the sum total of the assets that you have accumulated over your lifetime; that is, real estate, stocks, bonds, life insurance, and personal items.

Depending upon the size of your estate, your estate planning attorney might recommend forming a living trust.

If you are the parent of children under the age of eighteen, you will need to decide who will care for your children. You can name a guardian for your children in your will. If you are a single parent of minor children, you will want to discuss who to name as the guardian. Also, you may want to consider establishing a trust to look after their financial needs.

When you have a serious illness such as breast cancer, and you have minor children, it is recommended that you apply for Social Security benefits for you and your children. Children are eligible for Social Security benefits until their nineteenth birthday or if they are enrolled in college, whichever comes first.

 Fact

A living trust allows a trustee that you have appointed (attorney, accountant, or bank) to step in and manage your financial affairs.

Decide who you and your partner would choose to care for your children if you were both deceased so that both your input can be considered. If you are the one living with breast cancer, you may want to seek a full-time caregiver to care for your children early on so that your child will develop a relationship with his caregiver while you can still oversee and provide guidance to both. This is one way to help your caregiver instill the values that you feel are important while sharing your wisdom with them on the special needs of your child.

You may think that this is a morbid way to think, but you will alleviate many of the fears that keep you up at night, worrying about your children's future. In essence, you are replacing that fear with action and empowering yourself and your children by doing so.

It is the hope that your life goes on for many years and that you will be there for your children well into their adult years, but for now, you need to get the support for you, your spouse/partner, and your children. You can approach the issue of hiring a caregiver for your children early on as a support person for you and your family, integrating him or her into your family life and getting the help that you need while going through your treatments. Your caregiver can help with meal planning and with rides for the children and for yourself, and be your right arm (your assistant) to ease the stresses of managing your home life, work life, and personal life. After you complete your breast cancer treatments, then you can keep him or her on board to relieve you of some of your responsibilities so that you can spend more quality time with your children and the people you love.

When selecting a caregiver for your children, make sure that you ask questions about his or her morals and values, because this person will likely influence your children and you will want to make sure that his or her values complement the values and morals that you have instilled in them.

Make Plans—Expect to Live

You can live purposefully by identifying your life goals and live according to them. If you can live each day with the expectation that your life will go on, however many days lie ahead, each will be rich and purposeful. You can begin by actively preparing spiritually and developing your own personal relationship with God or another higher being. In addition, some other ways to achieve peace with what the future holds include:

- Find reasons to celebrate and view each day as an opportunity.
- Give to others by sharing yourself and your wisdom.
- Be sensitive to the messages of your body in relation to feelings of joy and stress.
- Listen to uplifting music.
- Laugh and play.
- Read uplifting books.
- Resolve issues that have interfered with your happiness.
- Upon awakening, try to be open to the possibilities that unfold before you.

Life is a gift: Affirm this gift within you as you go about your daily routines. The ordinary is the extraordinary once you have journeyed this path. You have been through a tiring journey—renew your spirit, be gentle with yourself, rest in the spirit, and be present to yourself, and a new life will be yours, a different life that is filled with a new appreciation for living. Be hopeful, as hope instills life and life breeds more life—the spiritual life that is within will bring you peace. Explore your inner spirit, your relationship with God or another higher being. This will set your life force free.

CHAPTER 16

Write Your Own Story

It is all about you. There is a gift that only you can give others and that is to share your personal story. The important thing about writing your own story is that it frees you to look at who you are and helps you to identify your feelings while reviewing your life. Your story is never just about you but also the people in your life who have shaped your likes and dislikes, happy times and regrets, values and disappointments, and many other aspects of your life as you know it and perceive it to be. This chapter will give you ideas on how to share your story and who to share it with. An outline of questions will be included to get you started as well as some ideas as to how to start this adventure.

Trace Your Family History; Create a Legacy

Creating a genealogy of your family by tracing your family roots helps you gain insight into who you are and where you came from. Create a legacy by writing your family background, traditions, and values. Compile pictures, videos, and special gifts that can be shared with the loved ones who will continue your legacy and remembrance in their own lives. Sharing words of wisdom—for example, at a special family celebration, perhaps your daughter's or son's wedding—or knitting a blanket to be given at your loved one's baby shower, are ways to create a legacy of memories that can be passed on for future generations.

There are so many creative ways to leave a legacy to those you love. Here are some ideas for you to think about:

- Organize and place your pictures in albums.
- Record audiotapes to be played with the photo albums.
- Keep a journal that you would like shared after your death.
- Designate any special jewelry, or collections to be given to family and friends.
- Write letters to the special people in your life.
- Write down special family memories to be shared.
- Express your love and encouragement to those who are a special part of your life.
- Write down favorite family recipes.
- Share your favorite books and children books.
- List your most memorable life's experiences and the wisdom you would like to pass on to your loved ones.

Plan a Family Reunion

Planning a celebration, whether for family, childhood friends, or friends from any memorable stage in your life, is a joyous gift to give yourself and your circle of support. If your family or a friend wants to help you with the reunion/celebration, let them help. Getting friends involved by having them tell you their favorite memory for you to compile and share at the party is a gift you can give to your guests.

Plan a creative family reunion. For example, if you are of Italian descent, plan for everyone to bring a favorite Italian dish that they remember from their childhood. If you are of Irish descent, you may want to have your reunion at an Irish cultural center or share old pictures of your ancestors, or better yet have the reunion in Ireland, or wherever your family roots began.

Write Letters to the Special People in Your Life

Preparing emotionally for living with breast cancer involves sharing special thoughts, values, and wisdom with your loved ones. These can be shared verbally or in writing, though the written word is more apt to have a lasting value. Writing down memories, hopes, and dreams with your loved ones frees you to be truly present with them now by giving you clarity on how your life has had meaning because of the other people in your life.

 Fact

> Another way to tell your story is to do an oral history of you and your family that you can share with the important people in your life. Depending on your technical abilities, you can even have someone you are comfortable with videotape you and capture those messages that you would like to give your children, and words of encouragement to those family and friends who have relied on you. You can be creative and do individual ones for those people you cherish.

The storytelling process is dependent on you and can be anything you want it to be. Some examples include creating personal gifts or simply writing down who you would like to pass your favorite possessions on to. These may include a favorite piece of jewelry, furniture, books, or a special collection that has brought you joy and you know just the person who would appreciate it and share your love and passion for it. In order to write to others, you first need to write your own story or at least ask yourself the questions and the messages that you would like to share. And only then can you share with others . . . the rest of the story.

Wisdom That You Would Like to Pass On

In all of life's experiences, wisdom is to be gained. Having been on the breast cancer journey and living with it, past, present, and future, brings wisdom that only is realized through suffering and the inner strength that is a result of the experience. The Bible says that wisdom comes from God, but in other teachings it can come through contemplative thought, the nature of life, or being present with one's thoughts and at peace with oneself, others, and the world.

Whatever your beliefs about wisdom, it is something that is deeply personal, profound, and not easily shaken from your constitution. Wisdom is often an insight gained from your experiences in life or in others' lives. Wisdom is not something that is controversial, but ingrained in the essence of your being. In other words, your wisdom is not to be reckoned with—it is not a point of debate—because it is formed by your personal thoughts and beliefs through what you have experienced.

Your life's wisdom is the most cherished gift that you can give those you love. Honor your own wisdom and share it with the special people in your life.

 Alert

Your wisdom is something that is to be honored and respected because it comes from your heart. It is the wisdom of your inner convictions that your loved ones will want to know about you. To pass on your wisdom is to pass on life itself. It empowers others to grow and it is told in a way that says, "This is what worked for me."

Family/Friend Traditions

Whatever your family's and friend's traditions, big or small, holiday or every day, they have special warm feelings that accompany them. Many traditions are based on a long history dating from previous generations that have been passed on just because that's what "they always have done." Many of those traditions have deep roots that may not even be fully understood by the present generation. Asking yourself about the traditions that you value most, and what they mean to you, and then sharing those memories will help present and future generations understand and perhaps carry on your favorite traditions.

⌶ Essential

Giving others the freedom to incorporate new family traditions that evolve from generation to generation can be fun and a creative way to adapt what worked in the past to meet the needs of the present. Not everyone comes from a family of rich traditions and some may be unconventional, but always they are uniquely yours.

For those who do not have family, there are always friends and significant others in your life that add meaning and joy that may even become traditions. For example, if you are single and have no immediate family, you can start a tradition of beginning your holiday season by watching a vintage movie with a friend, such as *Miracle on 34th Street*, or going out to a favorite restaurant during the holiday season. By doing this, you create new memories in your life. Some traditions, such as the Jewish Seder, already incorporate goodwill by inviting a stranger to the family table to celebrate Passover. You can always share your family traditions with others by writing down what they mean to you or just by living them with new meaning and appreciation.

Family Recipes

No matter what your ethnic background, you probably have many family recipes or special ways of cooking that you just do without thinking. Have you ever baked your mom's favorite cookies, the ones that remind you of your childhood? The smells in the kitchen, the taste in your mouth, and the fond memories of love and warmth will accompany the recipes that you write down for your children and succeeding generations, or perhaps share with other special people in your life. Writing the recipes down is one sure way to pass them on for others to enjoy. You can also give the recipe as a gift to go along with the tradition that it is associated with the baked goods.

Special Memories in Your Life

If you had to write about the three most cherished memories in your life, what would you choose to write about? The memories you pick tell a lot about what is important to you. You can choose memories from different stages in your life, i.e., childhood, young adulthood, or adulthood. The beauty of writing your own story is that there is no right or wrong. Depending on your life's experiences, your memories can vary from getting your first bike, graduating college, your parents' love, the birth of your child, or your very first job. It could be a memory of a person in your life that influenced you to be the person you are today.

Whatever you choose to write about, make sure that you are sensitive to those loved ones who will be reading your words. It is always best to write when you are in a position of strength and not feeling vulnerable. If you are living in the end stages of your illness, you want to be careful not to try to control your loved ones after you are gone. The message should be one of empowerment and love and one of teaching and encouragement. These words will be lasting in the hearts and minds of those you love.

How to Write the Story of Your Life

There are questions to ask and to explore, and you can invite your feelings, thoughts, joys, and fears to be your guides. Or you can ask these questions of the people in your life with whom you are most comfortable, including friends, partners, family, or colleagues.

The following list of questions is meant to be a beginning of your story, focusing on key topics and areas of your life such as personal, historical, favorite work, values, your concept of God and the world, your likes and dislikes, and wishes and dreams. How you use these questions will reveal the story of your life.

- What makes your heart happy?
- What is your family history and roots?
- What are your three favorite memories?
- What are your spiritual beliefs?
- What do you like the most (such as foods, things to do, hobbies, favorite possessions)?
- What are your least favorite things, or pet peeves?
- What are the wishes and dreams you hold for you and others that you love?
- What would you like the special people in your life to remember about you?
- What words of wisdom would you like to leave to some of the special people in your life? For example, if you were to leave notes to your spouse, partner, children, sister, brother, friend, or someone who has had a powerful impact on your life, what would they say?
- What are the three most important values you feel have guided most of your decisions and are integrated in your everyday life?
- Who is the one person who has influenced your life in a positive way?
- What is the most important wisdom that you received during or after your breast cancer treatment?
- What message do you have for others living with breast cancer? Will you explain it?

- What one word comes to mind when you reflect on your life?
- What are the three most treasured accomplishments in your life?
- What would you say to the world if you could leave one important message?
- What message would you leave to your loved ones that would help them live the life they deserve?

The rest is up to you—what questions you ask, what you decide you would like to share and leave for others to know about you, and what the special people in your life mean to you.

CHAPTER 17

Stages of Grief

Many have heard of Dr. Elisabeth Kübler-Ross, who was a pioneer in the care, support, and counseling of those terminal patients. Dr. Kübler-Ross explored grief and dying and is well known for her book *On Death and Dying,* in which she first described her classically regarded "Five Stages of Grief." You may be wondering why this focus on death and dying—you thought this was a book about living with breast cancer. The grieving process applies to personal trauma, a crisis, or a dramatic change that comes as a result of the breast cancer diagnosis. Dr. Kübler-Ross wrote, "It is only when we truly know and understand that we have a limited time on earth—and that we have no way of knowing when our time is up, that we will then begin to live each day to the fullest as if it was the only one we had."

The Grief Cycle

This chapter will examine the five stages of grief, otherwise known as the grief cycle model:

- Denial
- Anger
- Bargaining
- Depression
- Acceptance

The grief cycle model is only a guide. Each individual has to experience her own journey of coming to grips with the possibility of death and dying. Acceptance of this reality is what enables a person to cope. The grief cycle model is not a rigid series of events, but one that is fluid from stage to stage, not necessarily in any particular sequence. An individual might also get stuck in one stage or will revisit the various stages if not completed. A person's grief is an individual process and the grief cycle model helps a person to understand her own and other peoples' emotional reaction to grief. The journey that follows the diagnosis involves the emotions of denial, anger, bargaining, depression, and hopefully acceptance. Going through these stages of grief will assist a woman who has been through the breast cancer journey to truly live. Let's look at how the grief cycle applies to dealing with a person's reaction to being diagnosed with breast cancer.

Denial

A little denial goes a long way in its role of self-protection. However, denial without reality or living with a fantasyland perspective will only keep you stuck and unable to move forward in your breast cancer experience. Denial comes with the initial shock of the breast cancer diagnosis. It is during this initial stage that you experience disbelief when you are given the information presented to you by your health care professional, information that cannot be completely absorbed or dealt with in a rational way because of its emotional impact.

When your doctor tells you that you have breast cancer, you think she has made a terrible mistake, that this is not happening to you. It is inconceivable to you that you have breast cancer and the shock of it all is too overwhelming. This is when a little denial can help get you through the initial shock. Denial is also a coping mechanism for family and friends. You will find that when you call to tell your loved ones that you have breast cancer, they initially don't believe you and you may find them asking the same questions over and over in disbelief, hoping that they misunderstood you.

Alert

When others question your breast cancer diagnosis, you may find yourself wondering if it is, in fact, true. After all, it shouldn't be happening to you; or to anyone else, for that matter. Perhaps it is a big mistake, and the doctor mixed up your pathology report with someone else's. You of course have heard of this happening in some situations, and mistakes can happen, you tell yourself. This is also denial.

Their denial is what this stage is all about. It is about shock, disbelief, and the feeling that having breast cancer is not something that was in your plans and therefore just can't be. There must be a very big mistake. Denial is essential in the initial grief cycle and helps us to cope with anticipated loss. It could be fear of the loss of your hair, breast, reproductive years, and, most importantly, the possibility of the loss of your life. Denial is a self-protection mechanism that helps you to decipher and process the information at hand, that you have breast cancer. Denial can happen not only at the initial diagnosis, but throughout your cancer journey. If your prognosis is grave, denial can help with the day-to-day coping with the reality of your situation and help cope with the end-of-life issues that are confronting you.

Anger

This emotion usually occurs when an individual is feeling helpless and powerless. You say to yourself "Why me?" or "What did I do to deserve this?" Anger is depicted in many different ways, depending on how the individual deals emotionally with significant trauma in her personal life, especially in a life-threatening situation such as having breast cancer and what it all means. People have pre-conceived fears about cancer, and most know someone close who had cancer and either survived or lost his or her life to it. All of your previous experiences have an impact on your feelings and knowledge of what you can expect. However, these perceptions may not be accurate and now this is happening to you. You may react with anger at yourself, blaming yourself for getting cancer because of something you may have done wrong in the past or for not taking care of your health the way you should. There is always something you will come up with to blame yourself for. You may be relentless in the way you treat yourself by manifesting your anger in a self-tormenting, self-centered way. For friends and family, this is hard to watch and they may try to reason with you that you did not cause it and feel helpless in their efforts.

 Fact

You may have anger directed toward others. You may find yourself angry at life, God, the people you are closest to, the feelings of guilt that you have breast cancer, and angry that you can't do and care for others the way you would like. Feeling guilt that you have contemplated these negative thoughts against the very people whom you care about may even add to your anger.

Anger is not a rational feeling that can be explained, but it feels so real and it can rear its ugly head not only toward your family and friends, but also toward your doctor, health care professionals, or anyone who has come into your life since your breast cancer diagnosis. Anger can also be manifested in blaming yourself. In other words, if you did not go through that divorce, or if your family life had not been so dysfunctional, you may not have been so stressed, which compromised your immune system and started your body making breast cancer cells.

Though not rational, your thought process can go in every direction and your thoughts need to be given respect and time so you can sort through the anger and work things through. Getting stuck in this stage can be very sad for both you and for the important people around you and may alienate the support system that is so vital to your recovery. Let go of the anger and move forward. Too much energy is wasted in this stage, energy you will need for healing your body, mind, and spirit.

Bargaining

At times you may ruminate about what you could have done to prevent breast cancer, perhaps eating healthier foods, exercising more, and drinking less, or maybe if you were just a different type of person then stress would not have gotten the best of you. Whatever you did wrong you may say you want to change, because if you change it then just maybe you will not get breast cancer again.

You could be bargaining with your God, yourself, your doctor, or no one in particular. Perhaps you have not taken good care of yourself, you're overweight, you let everything bother you, and have let other people's problems become yours so much so that you may have lost your personal sense of self. Bargaining involves self-preservation and self-care, which is not to be confused with being selfish. Your bargaining chip may sound like this: "If I get through my breast cancer treatments and live, I will change my ways. I will eat healthier, exercise more, enjoy the simple things in life, and not fret over so many unimportant tasks that occupied my time and energy before I had breast cancer."

Sounds easy and this life change may last for some time post–breast cancer treatment, but slipping back to your old ways can be a subtle process. In order to sustain the insights gained, you need to be purposeful in your pursuit of the negotiating you have done with yourself. If you find yourself preoccupied with all the things that should have been and imagine all the things and events that will never be, you may need to seek professional help, because if this is not resolved it may affect your healing process. After all, life is one big bargain, a series of choices, so you need to keep moving forward.

Depression

When coping with death, grief, and loss, whether it is a loss of health, or a loss of your life as you know it to be, it is a natural process to feel sadness, regret, and depression. During breast cancer treatment, it could be the loss of hair that may trigger the true extent of your illness and the seriousness of its treatment. It may be the loss of your breasts or perhaps the reality that you may not be able to have children because breast cancer treatment has put you into early menopause that triggered your depression. Whatever may have precipitated it, you not only have the right to feel this way, but the depression is also a precursor of the acceptance that follows.

 In Her Own Words

When I found out I had breast cancer I lost it. I was a not a nice person to be around. Then I saw what it was doing to my family. I could not destroy them. I first found the lump on the day my first granddaughter was born. I never thought I would live to see her grow up. I had the lump removed by a wonderful doctor, I went through radiation, I prayed and prayed. I know I have been blessed, with the help of my family, friends, and my faith. Every day I thank God for His blessings.

—**Liz, age 74, 15-year survivor**

For many, depression comes before change. It is the knocking-down phase before the building up, or the beginning of acceptance that will help restructure one's life.

Depression can rob you of energy, immobilize you, and bring to mind all that is negative. Depression comes when you have reached rock bottom and there seems to be no way out. It is another phase that occurs right before change happens. Change usually takes place when individuals are in pain. The old saying in the gym of "no pain, no gain" has some relevance here and some depression should be allowed, experienced, accepted, and then put to rest. However if depression persists, you should seek the help of a mental health professional.

 Fact

> None of the stages of grief should be given a larger place than any other as you cope with breast cancer. All need to be worked through in your own time, your own way, and in your own sequence with the people you choose to be with you—this is your individual journey.

It is often said in psychology journals that depression is anger turned inward. It is that feeling of loneliness, helplessness, and fear that deprives your inner being of peace and harmony. When faced with a life-threatening illness such as breast cancer, it is understandable that it may create a feeling of being overwhelmed and depressed. Acknowledge it, be with it, and eventually be done with it. There is too much that needs to be done so that acceptance can begin and you can find your new life.

Acceptance

Grief and loss come to a resolution with acceptance and vary according to the person's situation. Time allows you to resolve the overwhelming range of feelings that arise with change and life's difficult challenges. The grieving process contributes to an individual's healing. And healing occurs when the loss becomes part of the person's set of life experiences. Accepting the fact that you are living with breast cancer will free you to move forward. The breast cancer experience has become integrated into your life and becomes your "new normal." It is important to realize that once you have entered into the acceptance process, you can revert back to some of the earlier feelings throughout your lifetime.

Grieving a loss is not a sequential or rigid process, but one that ebbs and flows. There is also no time limit to the grieving process and each person defines one's own healing period. Whether you refer to it as Kübler-Ross's stages of death and dying or the grief cycle that occurs with any significant loss or change, understanding the stages helps you to better cope with the experience. Knowledge of these five stages can help you better understand yourself as you move through them. Perhaps recognizing that you have become stuck in one stage will assist you in becoming unstuck and allow you to have the support and time that you need to go through the process in your own unique way.

Survival

Whether you have cycled through the grieving process with ease or with much difficulty, you are now heading into the survival mode of healing, the take-charge and empowered way of life. You recognize that there is light at the end of the tunnel and you can now reflect on certain principles that may have helped you in your own healing process.

First, recognizing behaviors that may hinder the healing process is one way that will help you stay on track on the road of healing and peace. Behaviors that do not foster the healing process include:

- Avoiding or minimizing your emotions
- Use of excessive alcohol or drugs to self-medicate
- Losing yourself in work, whether a job, a hobby, or anything that occupies your time and energy so as to avoid dealing with your feelings

Survival tips that promote the healing process include:

- Give yourself time to experience your thoughts and feelings openly to yourself.
- Accept and acknowledge both positive and negative feelings.
- Journal your feelings to give clarity to them as you heal.
- Express your feelings openly to a trusted friend to share the significance of the losses in your life.
- Allow yourself the privilege of crying. It is a release that can free you of the overwhelming feelings that occur in the healing process.
- Reflect on your life and any unresolved business and try to come to a place of peace.
- Make a gratitude list of all that you have in your life to be thankful for.
- Participate in a breast cancer support group to share your experiences with others who understand.
- Seek professional help if you find that you are stuck and feeling too overwhelmed.

CHAPTER 18

Riding the Waves

Dealing with breast cancer is kind of like riding across the ocean in a sailboat. This chapter will teach you how to navigate life with the wind at your back and the horizon before you. Your goals are ahead, waiting to be discovered. A new adventure awaits you. How you choose to get to your destination (whatever it is to you) and what you find when you arrive there is up to you. It is not the destination that is important, but the journey.

Riding the Ups and Downs

When you think of your breast cancer experience, it seems like it is a series of ups and downs and just when you are getting comfortable, something happens, changing the course that you have strategically outlined. For example, you are on your next-to-the-last chemotherapy treatment and your doctor tells you that you cannot get the treatment until your blood counts are better. Your immediate reaction is, "No way, I have everything timed out so that when my treatments are over, I'm going on a vacation," or "I wanted to be done with my chemotherapy treatments before the holidays." You wonder how not having chemotherapy treatment can be so upsetting. It may temporarily take the wind out of your sails. But in time it all seems to work out and you are back on course. This is just one of the many ups and downs that happen during breast cancer treatment. So be well-prepared, stay on course, expect the unexpected. Learning to ride the waves is your new full-time job.

Fact

Many other unexpected events may occur during your cancer journey that put you in an emotional flurry, such as the day you find clumps of your hair everywhere. A mouth sore develops or a vaginal infection flares up because your immune system is compromised from your breast cancer treatment. Or you look in the mirror and you don't even recognize yourself. These are just some of the ups and downs that make staying on course so challenging.

The Ups

What could possibly be an up during this time of overwhelming challenges? After all, you have breast cancer. Finding the ups in down time means taking a telescopic view. But once you realize that, you will find there are benefits to going through breast cancer treatment.

In Her Own Words

Choose hope. Treat hope as an art to develop and to practice. Nurture it and then use it as a gift to another woman facing a difficult part of the breast cancer journey. Your true healing is connected to gifting this art.

—Mary Pat, age 61, 7-year survivor

It may be a kindness extended to you by a friend or total stranger at a time you need it most. It may be the first time in your life that you realize how much people really care about you. The experience certainly puts another dimension into your life and perspective, one where you may have even learned to live more joyfully. The ups are whatever you define them to be. Perhaps a newfound wisdom, an insight, and a deeper understanding of the importance of your relationships and choices you make. An upside of your breast cancer experience could also be the peace that you have never been able to successfully achieve with a past relationship or circumstance in your life. You finally have simplified your life, the sun is shining, and you are feeling strong enough to set your own sails.

The Downs

You are sailing through your breast cancer treatments and all of a sudden there is a dark and stormy spell. Nothing seems to be going right. Your doctor is recommending another test to see how your chemotherapy treatments are working. You wonder, what does this all mean? You may just be having a bad wig day and you feel like everyone is staring at you and wondering why you look so different. People who may not know that you are undergoing breast cancer treatment may secretly be saying, "What did she do to her hair?"

Many of the downs happen unintentionally, such as the feeling of disappointment you may have in people who have not been sensitive to your needs and are uncomfortable being with you because of your cancer. They may have some faulty thinking about cancer and its treatment and because of this, are ill-equipped to support you. It is important to remember that you may not have the energy or the strength to educate others and you must carefully choose where to invest your energy resources.

The Calm

You finally have gotten into the rhythm of your new life after breast cancer treatment and you are settling in. The ups and downs don't seem so extreme and you find yourself sailing along with the ebb and flow of your daily life with breast cancer. You now at least know what and expect. There are fewer surprises and yes, you have become somewhat of an expert sailor when it comes to managing it all. At times, you even surprise yourself by how far you have come in your journey.

Having breast cancer has sunk into your mind, body, and spirit, and you are determined not to go down with the ship. It brings about a serene sense of calm that at times feels foreign. You ask, "Am I on another planet?" Or maybe the acceptance stage that you are in now is helping you let go and center your life in the present. You have learned to find peace in the midst of adversity, a navigating skill that can only be acquired through experience and the choices you make.

The Storm

You finally think things are going well, you are getting used to the idea that you can find a sense of calm even for a brief moment, and then a storm hits.

You plant your feet firmly on the deck and begin the fight of your life as a long series of turbulent waves hit and you don't even have time to think or rest. It could be an infection that lands you at a hospital or a deep depression that takes you off to a far remote place that seems to offer no way back. This is when all the previous ups and downs that you have experienced just don't compare. But you have learned some tips along the way and they can help you navigate your way back to calmer seas.

As with all storms, an end is certain and how you choose to navigate with weather conditions will safely get you to port.

Weathering the Storm

Sailing through life is not about the size of the sailboat you have, or the equipment you own. It's about being a resourceful captain and steward of your boat, its resources, the people you choose to have along on your journey, and where you allow yourself to go.

It is learning to ride the waves. Weathering the storm makes you strong, durable, flexible, and more resilient. Experience makes you an expert sailor. You become stronger, wise, and always more prepared for the unexpected. Becoming an expert sailor requires you to learn new techniques, come through some rough storms, and then lets you enjoy the peaceful and serene times that also become part of the sailing experience, where you glide with the breeze, enjoying the nature around you. A novice sailor may be energetic, and have the best boat and the newest equipment, but the seasoned sailor brings the depth that adds value and wisdom to the voyage.

Essential

When you are at the start of the breast cancer journey, you can join hands with other shipmates who have been through the breast cancer experience to strengthen your position. There is less of a chance the ship will capsize if there is a good solid crew, so learn to let others help, take in their wisdom, and sail your boat in only the way that you can—with grace and courage.

Navigating It All

As you learn to ride the waves, the ups, the downs, the calm and the storm, it then becomes easier for you to stay on course. Aim for your destination and keep your eyes on the horizon. Was there a visit to your family's ancestral home, a trip you always postponed because of other people's needs? Or maybe that sports car or sailboat you always wanted but just couldn't justify the cost? Well now you can. Navigating this requires you to be completely present in all you do and having breast cancer has become a means to an end that really is a true beginning of the rest of your life.

CHAPTER 19

When Someone You Love Is Diagnosed with Breast Cancer

If you are the support person for someone who is experiencing the emotional upheaval of breast cancer, knowing how to deal with feelings that surface while helping your loved one will have a positive impact on her recovery. An important part of being there for someone is recognizing that it might bring up your own feelings of loss. This chapter will explore some of the feelings and frustrations that come up when caring for a loved one with breast cancer. Some general guidelines and tips will be covered, but the specifics of how to help are always up to the individual. Being creative in helping your loved one is best when it comes from your heart.

Your Role as Supporter

The first thing that comes to mind when a close friend or loved one has been diagnosed with breast cancer is, "What can I do to help?" Then the realization sets in that there is no book to read, thing to buy, or gift to give that can make things better for either the person with breast cancer or you, the support person. It is at times a lonely journey, even with all the supports available. And for the support person, the confidant, it can also be lonely not knowing what to do or say. These feelings are often overwhelming for someone who has not dealt with them before.

Coping with Feelings of Helplessness

The support person goes through his or her own grieving process and feels vulnerable while trying to be there to support his or her loved one. It is a tough job, but an important role that comes with a sense of great responsibility. A true support person understands the loved one's needs and coping strategies based on knowledge of what has helped from shared experiences. You will be there through each stage of breast cancer treatment, helping deal with the emotional upheaval that occurs. But sometimes it just doesn't feel like you are doing enough.

Essential

Researchers have reported that when patients go to their appointments they hear only one-tenth of what is being said—especially in the early diagnostic period—because the tendency is to focus on the emotional impact, their jobs, and their family responsibilities. One big way to support your loved one is to offer to accompany her to her doctor appointments and take notes or just listen and verify what was said.

Communicating with a loved one going through treatment and expressing your concerns to her is part of the ongoing friendship and trust that has already been established. Her breast cancer will add another dimension to the relationship and will solidify the bond. Feeling helpless and being present for someone are two different aspects of the cancer experience as well as in the support process.

There is no one standard way to communicate and express your own concerns as the support person. This answer is based on each individual's approach to any kind of crisis. When you are the support person, there will be times that you will have to keep your concerns to yourself or find someone else with whom you can share these concerns. The important thing is not to add more of a burden to your loved one, who is already struggling to keep things together.

If coping with these feelings of helplessness becomes overwhelming, there are always caregiver support groups that you may want to join, or professional help may be available at the local cancer center where your loved one is getting her treatments. You may also choose to seek individual counseling on this matter if needed.

In Her Own Words

I felt that my part in my friend's life during her battle with breast cancer was to validate. Validate that everything about it sucked. When your friend is faced with having both her breasts removed—instead of saying "Just cut them off, get rid of them"—it's okay to say "This sucks!" Validate that it's okay to not be happy and perky all the time, just to make everyone else feel okay; it's okay to cry.

—Beth, age 53, friend

Coping with feelings of helplessness is a common occurrence for both the person with breast cancer as well as the support person. Recognizing that this is a common bond between you will also help in the coping process.

Alert

Do not be of false cheer, saying to your loved one, "Don't worry, everything will turn out okay." This may be helpful for a split second, but then reality sets in and it may just add to their stress. It is better to say, "I am here for you."

The Best Person for the Job
Overshadowing it all is that feeling that you are a helpless bystander and there must be something you could be doing to make it better. After all, she is depending on you for support. The

role of the support person is one of utmost respect and honor and you have been specially chosen for this role. You take this responsibility seriously because it is a role that only you can fulfill. Go with confidence, letting go of that feeling of helplessness and the need to make it all better. Even though you are sailing in unknown territory, recognize that you know her the best and can draw on those shared past experiences and simply walk beside her.

If you are not sure about your own sense of strength in coping with your loved one's breast cancer experience and are focused on what her illness will mean to you, be patient. You are going through the process along with her. You will need to ground yourself in the past experiences that you have shared with her, remembering how you were able to work through them triumphantly. All this will help you move forward with the needed strength that will sustain the two of you throughout the experience.

 Alert

If you are not chosen to do a certain task that you have offered, it is important to not take it personally. Remember the answer is always to make the journey as manageable as possible and follow your loved one's lead.

A good rule of thumb to use to evaluate whether you are the best person for the job is to find out your loved one's level of need for support. Does your loved one want to listen to your concerns and console you? This may provide a distraction for her, but it probably will be short lived. Does bringing up the subject of anxious feelings about this journey to your loved one provide her with relief at knowing that the subject is out in the open, or does bringing up your concerns add anxiety and fear to your loved one who is already burdened from breast cancer treatment and other adjustments needed to get through treatment? If you, the support person, cannot identify the best approach, you may want to consult with professionals. Seek the help of the social worker or psychologist at your local breast cancer center for support.

However, if you feel you are not the best person for the job, perhaps you can help identify and approach another person who may be better at meeting her emotional needs. You can still help by organizing and scheduling rides for treatment or doctor appointments, or you could offer to shop for groceries and do errands while another support person is the "listen to feelings" person. The fact that you are asking to help shows your concern and willingness to be there for her.

How Can You Help Your Loved One During Breast Cancer Treatment?

There are so many ways to help. The following is the short list of options to help trigger your instincts and creativity and help you support your loved one during breast cancer treatment.

- Provide rides to chemotherapy or radiation treatments.
- Make a meal for your friend or her family, but be sensitive to the side effects one experiences during cancer treatments. Avoid heavy gravy on meats and rich foods that may upset her stomach, and foods that are not easily digested.
- Go to a doctor appointment to be a second set of ears.
- Go along for a massage, a car ride, time at the beach, or whatever your loved one's favorite activity. This will help you both with a feeling of normalcy during treatments
- Be outrageous! Give your loved one permission to be outrageous. Suggest a do-rag instead of a wig, go on a motorcycle ride if she is up to it, or plan a weekend away and tell her that the weekend is a special weekend for her.
- Celebrate significant dates during breast cancer treatment. For example, help plan a party to celebrate the final

chemotherapy treatment for her, but make sure she doesn't do all the work.

- Celebrate all important milestones, years after her breast cancer treatment. For example, have a pizza party on her fifth year of living with breast cancer and invite all the people that helped her get through her treatments.
- Allow your relationship to grow and change, and be there and just listen. You may be the only one that she can talk to and with whom she is comfortable talking about what is really on her mind.
- Just be there, be present and available to her.

Share Your Talents

Talents can include the ability to help and to comfort, as well as to express yourself to others and the world. Your unique talent, whether it is one of comfort—adding light and humor to life, organizing, taking charge, or quietly listening, is the best thing to share with a loved one going through breast cancer treatment.

You may be a talented cook, a baker, a gardener, or a painter, to mention just a few areas that can bring great joy to a friend or loved one who is going through treatment. You may be the person who helps your loved one deal with the multitude of medical bills, helping to organize this daunting task when there are so many other daily life changes confronting her. Be creative and openly communicate with your loved one and share your special talents and make new memories to cherish in this most difficult time in both your lives.

Do Everything Out of Love

It is important to remember that whatever you do as a result of love is usually recognized. Even if you feel you have said or done the wrong thing, people are usually very forgiving when that thing has been done with good intentions. People are not experts at what to do for their loved ones when they have breast cancer and it probably is the first time that you have had to deal with such an illness. But if you have a good relationship with your loved one you could simply ask, "What can I do to help?" Knowing that perhaps there is nothing you can do, other than the fact that you are genuinely concerned, is at times just what the doctor ordered.

Extending a kindness by sending a card just to let her know you are thinking about her is one thing you can do when the person is not receptive to having you doing anything or helping in any way. Just reaching out is a positive thing that you can do and is appreciated by someone who is dealing with breast cancer treatments. Respect the fact that your role may be that of a bystander, ready to help as your loved one decides who will help her with what. Recognize that some individuals have a difficult time accepting help—as they are much more comfortable giving than receiving help from others. Just because they have breast cancer doesn't change who they are. Being aware of her personality and your past experience with her will allow you to help in the right way, which is always out of love.

What if She Rejects My Help?

The focus is always to support your loved one going through breast cancer treatment, completing her treatments, and in the aftermath of the whole experience. If you remember this and do not personalize any rejection of your kind gestures, it will help you as the support person. There may be instances in which your loved one feels that your presence triggers deep emotional feelings. She may not be ready to deal with these feelings and this may be a reason for rejecting your help. This may even be a subconscious thought and she may not be aware of why she does not want your help. But she will also know that your feelings are hurt. You may want to reassure her that whatever works for her, you will support. By offering your assistance, she will know that you care and that may simply be all that is needed from you.

In Her Own Words

One of my most painful memories is the day I met my friend at the supermarket, after several weeks of her not taking or returning my calls and not accepting a visit. I knew she was in a deep, dark place and I wanted to help, but she was not ready to receive it. In the dairy aisle, I hardly recognized my friend, who had lost her hair but had not yet purchased a wig. As soon as she saw me, I was thrilled to hear her say, "Why don't you come over to the house later?" After that, we talked, visited, and lamented. It was great to return to our regular, frequent contacts as friends.

—Marie, age 54, friend

Follow Your Heart and Be There for Her

When caring for someone with breast cancer, understand that your intuition and heart will speak to you and help you decide what is best to do for your loved one. Caring for others is not an exact science with dos and don'ts, but only a gut feeling of what one should do in the face of illness and how to reach out to someone you love. Being in tune with your gut and your heart will assist you in the discovery of how to help your loved one. It may be a trial and error approach but one that will work as long as you listen to your heart.

Being present for someone, and being flexible and available to help in any way that your loved one has requested or accepted from you is the best way to ease the pain. Walking alongside that person and just saying to your loved one that you will be there for her is the best way to show your love and concern. Being genuine in your approach to help with your heartfelt efforts will be appreciated by those who are going through the breast cancer journey. Be cautious not to be of false cheer—that is not what your loved one is seeking. She simply wants the support, love, and caring expressions that only you can give. Be generous with your time and ability to serve during this time and it will strengthen the bond with your loved one and give you the inner peace of knowing that you have made the road a little easier for your loved one during her breast cancer journey.

If Your Mother, Sister, Aunt, or Grandmother Is Diagnosed

Once a close relative is diagnosed with breast cancer, there is the immediate fear that arises that one day you, too, may be diagnosed with breast cancer. This is a legitimate and natural question and concern for anyone who is a close family member. Do not be ashamed of these feelings. You should first consult with your doctor and make sure you are up to date with your screening mammograms. Let your doctor know about your family member who has been diagnosed with breast cancer. This will make him aware of your situation and the anxiety that you may be feeling. Recognize that you may be at a higher risk for getting breast cancer and that you will need to be diligent about your breast health care and needs.

 Fact

Dealing with the fear of someday being diagnosed with the disease follows the same path as being diagnosed with the disease. First, you need to seek information and educate yourself about your personal risk of getting breast cancer. You may want to seek genetic counseling depending on your loved one's breast cancer diagnosis and characteristics. Many breast cancer centers have a high-risk screening program that you may want to participate in.

In the same way as your close family member made her personal choice about treatment based on her treatment options, you will have to make a personal choice. For example, your sister may have opted for a bilateral prophylactic mastectomy as her choice for treatment once she discovered her high risk and genetic predisposition for recurrence. You will need to examine your own genetic predisposition by seeking genetic counseling, or choose to keep a careful watch and be diligent about breast cancer screening and self-breast exams. It is important to know that whatever you choose, it should be an informed decision. Knowledge will make for better decisions, especially when it is a life-sustaining decision with many physical and emotional implications.

CHAPTER 20

What's New in Breast Cancer Research and Treatment

Our hope for the future lies in research. Research covers all areas of breast cancer, from its causes and its prevention to its treatment. The keys to the future should involve improved prevention, easier diagnosis, more precise categorization of types (threatening versus nonthreatening cancers), and better treatments. The major problem with preventing breast cancer is that we are not yet very good at identifying who will and who won't get it. The good news is that these days changes come fast in breast cancer research. The ultimate hope lies not in the cure of breast cancer, but in breast cancer prevention. For now, it is exciting to learn that new trends and clinical treatments that more accurately target certain kinds of cancer are available, and that new clinical trials of an experimental breast cancer vaccine were expected to begin in the spring of 2009.

The Present

Breast cancer research studies the factors that influence the cancer's development and looks at new ways to detect breast cancer and improve how it is diagnosed. Mammography remains the gold standard for screening, but thousands of women need to be screened in order to prevent one cancer death. Mammography may not be very efficient, and better screening tests are needed.

Breast center treatments and the use of new chemotherapy combinations also get a lot of attention. One of the most complex areas to understand is stem cell research, which looks at a cancer cell's microbiology and gene makeup to better predict which women will benefit from adjuvant chemotherapy. Examining cancer cells under a microscope with the goal of finding newer ways of looking at how the cells of a tumor are composed will help to predict the aggressive properties of the tumor, thus helping to guide a treatment course.

 Fact

> The more that is known about your breast cancer tumor, the better able you will be to choose your treatment of choice. Determining the properties that make up your breast cancer, such as estrogen/progesterone status and HER-2 status, will help tailor the treatment you get from your health care team (surgeons, radiologist, and oncologist).

This chapter will look at how two newer gene tests—Oncotype DX and MammaPrint—work, and how to request, understand, and interpret these tests and review their limitations. Also, it will include an explanation of what translational research is and how it can make more of an immediate contribution in breast cancer treatment as it swiftly translates research conclusions from lab to patient.

What kind of impact breast cancer treatment has on quality of life is also an area of study. For many years, scientists and helping professions have been studying the effects of treatment decisions and what impact those effects have on the quality of a patient's life. Research in this area can give insight to both medical professionals and individuals going through breast cancer treatment.

What impact our environment has on breast cancer and how it promotes it has also been an area of concern. The greening of America and the rest of the globe is of interest to everyone, not only those with the early onset of breast cancer. The commitment to research can help lead to breast cancer prevention. It relates to all levels of breast cancer—how cancer cells are made, how they spread to other organs, the drugs that interfere with cancer's growth, and the environment both in our bodies and the world in which we live. Preventing breast cancer may seem like a lofty goal, but it is one that has its roots in the beauty of humankind, and rests on the virtues of commitment to and love for ourselves, and our world.

New Chemotherapy Combinations and Treatments

Different combinations of treatment for early-stage breast cancers are now being studied. A new combination of chemotherapy drugs, Taxotere and Cytoxan (or TC), works as well as the standard Adriamycin and Cytoxan, and is easier on the heart, according to a recent study. TC is being used in early stage breast cancer patients who are at high risk for recurrence. Its effectiveness is still being investigated.

 Fact

In the April 2009 issue of the *New England Journal of Medicine*, a study indicated that Taxol, given weekly, improved disease-free survival rates and Taxotere, given every three weeks, showed improved survival. Later studies showed Taxol given after Adriamycin and Cytoxan only helped patients whose tumors were HER-2 positive or estrogen-receptor negative, and did little to tumors that were HER-2 negative and estrogen-receptor positive.

Studies suggest that hormone therapies, such as tamoxifen and raloxifene, which cut off the supply of estrogen to tumors that are receptive to the hormone, lower the risk for developing breast cancer in postmenopausal women.

Newer drugs called aromatase inhibitors—Arimidex (anastrozole), Aromasin (exemestane), and Femara (letrozole)—are being looked at to see if they, too, can fight estrogen-sensitive cancers. These drugs are currently being used to prevent cancer recurrence in an adjuvant role.

Dose-dense chemotherapy is also being researched. This is what it sounds like—giving chemotherapy more often. In this study, it's every two weeks, as opposed to the usual every-three-weeks dosing, to see if it works better in preventing recurrence. Clinical trials are underway to study the role of dose-dense chemotherapy in adjuvant situations.

Patient participation in clinical trials will advance breast cancer treatment options by allowing newer drugs and combinations of drug therapies to be studied.

New Therapeutic Advancements— Precision Guided Cancer Treatment

Gene expression tests to help with treatment decisions are now available to women who have early-stage breast cancer. These tests identify whether a woman's tumor has an aggressive nature and therefore has a higher risk of recurring. Adjuvant chemotherapy decisions are now made easier by the recent development of the Oncotype DX and MammaPrint gene tests, which help weigh the benefits against the risks of chemotherapy for early-stage breast cancer. The tests work by measuring a woman's risk for recurrence by analyzing whether her gene expression patterns show she is more susceptible to aggressive cancers that are more likely to spread to distant sites in the body.

The tests help to refine the risk of recurrence with early stage breast cancer in estrogen receptor positive and node negative tumors, and have only been approved and used in recent years.

The Oncotype DX test analyzes a panel of twenty-one cancer genes from a small piece of tissue removed during surgery. This analysis helps determine the tumor's chance of coming back after treatment. It scores recurrence as low risk (1–17), intermediate risk (16–30), or high risk with (a score of 31 or above). The highest score possible is 100. Those with a low risk would receive no or little benefit from chemotherapy treatment and the benefit isn't clear for the intermediate-risk group. But for the high-risk group, where recurrence is likely, the benefit of chemotherapy significantly outweighs the risk.

The MammaPrint was approved last year by the Food and Drug Administration (FDA) and looks at 70 genes in a breast tissue sample that has been surgically removed. A clinical trial in Europe called MINDACT (Microarray In Node-negative Disease may Avoid Chemotherapy Treatment) is underway to study its use in the clinic. However, it requires fresh tissue, so it will likely never be used in the United States.

It is important to note that the use of molecular signatures, which is what is tested with the Oncotype DX test, is just starting. Some think this approach will be the future. At some point, we may be able to decide on the prognosis of a tumor and how effective treatment will be by using molecular typing of cancers rather than relying on traditional staging.

 ## In Her Own Words

Amazing progress has been made over the last ten years, thanks to funding, brilliant scientists, and patients willing to be in clinical trials. I'm in a clinical trial because I want to be part of scientific advancement, and have a great deal of hope due to the dedication I see in the medical community to keep exploring new treatments.

—Nanci, age 55, 1-year survivor

Those women found to be at an intermediate risk will have another tool available to help refine their decision for adjuvant chemotherapy called TAILORx (Trial Assigning Individualized Options for Treatment). This study is sponsored by the National Cancer Institute (NCI) and will be available in several more years.

Targeted therapies are a classification of newer drugs that respond to specific gene changes that cause cancer.

Newer Imaging Tests

There are two recent developments in new imaging methods that are now being studied to detect breast cancers, especially in younger women who have denser breasts. Molecular breast imaging (MBI) is a technique that uses a special camera along with traditional mammography. Early studies presented at the Era of Hope meeting (which showcases new research findings supported by the Department of Defense Breast Cancer Research Project) suggested that it may be about as accurate as more expensive magnetic resonance imaging (MRI) and costs only $500.

Tomosynthesis (3D mammography) is an extension of digital mammography. The woman lies down on a table, her breast hangs through a hole, and the x-ray machine rotates around the breast to show a three-dimensional picture. This method is considered experimental and may help identify smaller tumors that may not be found with standard mammography.

Radiation Therapy

Recently, two newer radiation therapy techniques have been used offering a more convenient schedule, with larger daily doses. One is hypofractionated radiation, in which radiologists give a larger dose of radiation over a few days with an overall radiation plan of three weeks, as opposed to the standard five-week plan. Other studies are looking at shortening the time even more.

Accelerated partial breast irradiation (APBI), another technique that minimizes the amount of radiation affecting normal tissue with a more targeted approach, is also being studied.

HER-2 Targeted Therapies

Drugs that target HER-2 (a gene that produces a protein that helps cancer grow), such as Herceptin (trastuzumab) and Tykerb (lapatinils), work by preventing the protein from helping breast cancer cells divide. They also help the immune system fight the protein's growth. This type of gene affects about 20 to 25 percent of patients. Tykerb is a pill recently approved by the FDA for this cancer when it is advanced and cancer cells have not responded to Herceptin.

Many of the drugs for this type of cancer were first approved for metastatic disease and then tested for use in early-stage disease. Other drugs are being tested that target the same protein. With all the different types of drugs available for different types of cancer, Adjuvant! Online is an Internet program that can help you make an early stage breast cancer treatment decision.

Anti-angiogenesis Drugs

Anti-angiogenesis drugs are used to cut the blood supply that feeds cancer cells. An example of an anti-angiogenesis drug is Avastin (bevacizumab). There are some studies that have found that breast cancers surrounded by many new blood vessels are likely to be more aggressive. This is an area of research that needs further study before the theory can be validated.

One new discovery that shows promise, outlined in the January 2009 *Cancer Cell*, is the gene metaherin (also known as MTDH), which is found to be responsible for the aggressive nature of some tumors. Those tumors that express MTDH tend to be more resistant to chemotherapy and more likely to spread to other organs. Now that the gene has been identified, new drugs can be developed to counteract metaherin and prevent the cancer from spreading.

EGFR Targeted Drugs

Other drugs being worked on are those that target the epidermal growth factor receptor (EGFR) protein that is found in high amounts on the surface of some cancer cells. Two drugs that target EGFR, cetuximab (Erbitux) and eriotinib (Tarceva), are currently being used to treat other cancers. Studies are now looking at whether these drugs could also be used against breast cancers.

Biphosphonates

Biphosphonates are drugs used to reduce the risk of fractures in bones that have been weakened by metastatic disease. These drugs include pamidronate (Aredia) and zoledronic acid (zometa). The combination of hormone therapy and bisphosphonates is being studied for its treatment in early-stage breast cancer and its effect on reducing breast cancer risk.

Vitamin D

There has recently been a study involving vitamin D and its relationship to early-stage breast cancer. The study suggested that women deficient in vitamin D had a poorer outcome with their cancer treatments. More research is needed in the study of vitamin D, but it is an area that should be brought up with your doctor. Vitamin D supplements can also be helpful in preventing bone loss.

Breast Cancer Stem Cell Research

Following in the footsteps of the success of the human genome project, which mapped DNA and the genes of all human cancers, is the challenge of stem cell research. The human genome project helped scientists decode the 20,000 genes of the human genome, looking at specific mutations of cells and how they form malignant cancer cells. Can you imagine how knowing the genetic makeup of an individual's cancer cells and their response to drugs would have an impact on the treatment and hope for breast cancer's cure?

Researchers have already reported the gene profile of glioblastoma in brain cancer. Once these genomes are discovered, targeted new therapies can be developed.

Research studies on stem cells look at a cell's natural inclination to self-destruct. This self-destruction happens when it senses changes in the DNA structure in the cell and is part of the body's natural defense mechanism. Cell death is the way the body tries to rid itself of faulty cells so they won't grow back. The cancer stem cell theory purports that in tumor cells, there may be a small percentage of stem cells that are at the central core of cancer cells that are the most deadly. Many cancer therapies attack only tumor cells without destroying its stem cells. This will temporarily shrink a tumor, but it is the remaining stem cell that helps the tumor to regenerate. The goal in cancer stem cell research is to eradicate the cancer stem cells so that the tumor will not be able to continue growing.

The complexity and challenge of stem cell research is that these cells look different from patient to patient. To understand stem cells in breast cancer, you have to also look at the environment of normal healthy cells that surround it. How does one person have a body that is friendly to breast cancer cells and allows them to grow and another person's immune system kicks in to fight and destroy breast cancer cells? Researchers are trying to find an answer to that question. The goal is to stop breast cancer cells from traveling to other organs and sites. Knowing more about the microbiology of breast cancer stem cells will help researchers to target those mechanisms with new drugs before they take up residence in other parts of the body. Early detection along with advances in stem cell research and treatment gives a glimmer of new hope in the fight against breast cancer.

Quality of Life Research

Historically, the focus in breast cancer research was mainly on the scientific level, looking at the causes, growth, and treatment of breast cancer. Over the last fifteen years quality of life concerns have been researched—especially how quality of life has an impact on one's decision-making process in breast cancer treatment. Survivorship is also an area that is being studied, but is a relatively young research area. It is estimated that there are 12 million cancer survivors in the country today. Because of early detection, breast cancer affects a younger population, which makes make up a good number of cancer survivors.

Research is needed in survivorship issues that address quality of life, looking at the long- and short-term side effects of breast cancer treatment. Many of the long-term side effects, such as risks associated with chemotherapy and radiation treatments like early onset of menopause, fatigue, lymphedema, change in body image, fear of recurrence, and cognitive changes, linger on long after breast cancer treatment is over. Not only are there physical changes, but there are also the emotional and psychological impacts on the individual with breast cancer and the relationship with her caregivers.

In His Own Words

My wife and so many like her are called "survivors" for a reason. Surviving draws on the inner strengths of the victim and her loved ones. The chemo, radiation, and drugs that follow aren't easy, but they are successful. Each generation of ladies with the disease has better treatment options and greater hope thanks to the courage and perseverance of those who have survived before.

—Ward, husband of Ellen, 12-year survivor

Research of quality of life issues as they relate to breast cancer is also important. This knowledge will lead to the development of intervention early on in breast cancer treatment that will help ease the emotional upheaval by providing the medical professionals insight into how to help survivors adjust to life after breast cancer treatment. Other areas such as work re-entry, and diet and lifestyle changes can also help to educate breast cancer survivors on what to expect with treatment and help women be proactive in their quality of life choices during and after treatment.

Breast Cancer Vaccines Targeting HER-2 Breast Cancer

A vaccine, as well as new therapy, involving a vaccine to prevent the recurrence of positive cancer HER-2 began in spring 2009. The trial was given to 165 breast cancer patients with HER-2 tumors and lymph node involvement: 94 were vaccinated and 71 served as the control group and were not vaccinated. Researchers at Brooke Army Medical Center, San Antonio, Texas, are having some success in vaccinating breast cancer patients against its recurrence. The Neu Vax vaccine also known as (E75) is being used to test early-stage, HER-2 positive breast cancer. The study is small with a trial of 165 breast cancer patients, and after two-and-a-half years, the vaccinated group had both a lower risk of recurrence and was twice as likely to survive. The next trial, which may involve more than 700 patients, could offer the hope that women and researchers are striving for by providing better odds for women with HER-2 positive breast cancer. For now, it is still considered experimental and still too early to be considered conclusive, but is certainly a breakthrough that offers hope.

What Is Translational Research?

In translational research, results travel rapidly from the research lab, through clinical trials, and on to patients at a much faster pace than traditional research. Scientists, researchers, and doctors all work in concert to quickly get what's found out in the lab to the point where it can start making people well. It's frequently referred to as "bench to bedside" research, the bench being the lab, the bedside meaning treatment centers. The discoveries that begin at "the bench" are research at the most basic molecular or cellular level. Eventually, those findings are tested and then used on cancer patients. The goal of the process is a quick real-life response to what is discovered in the lab and relies on a coordinated approach with all the disciplines involved, such as microbiology and epidemiology.

Fact

> A consortium called Clinical and Translational Science Awards (CTSA) brings together academic health centers throughout the nation for the purpose of forming an interdisciplinary approach of investigators and research teams to promote innovative research that could be used in the front lines of clinical practice.

Translational research is often not funded by pharmaceutical companies or other private sources and relies on grants. Breast cancer is considered a varied illness with many different behaviors and characteristics. It takes many different kinds of scientists and researchers to look at these differences with the goal of combining efforts to complete clinical trials in a timely and successful manner through sharing of specimens, basic research, and working together for the goal of prevention and cure.

Essential

> In the fall of 2008, the three major U.S. television networks—CBS, ABC, and NBC—joined to raise money for traditional research with a nationwide telethon. The "Stand Up to Cancer" telethon raised more than $100 million. This brought an increased awareness to the importance of research and for out-of-the-box thinking with a vision of finding a cure.

With research funding being compromised during hard economic times, translational research efforts move fast at a lower cost than traditional research. One new discovery is the development of the drug Herceptin, which targets the cancer-friendly HER-2 protein. Development of this drug was made possible by an innovative translational research award from the Department of Defense Breast Cancer Research Program (BCRP) led by Dr. Dennis Slamon of UCLA's Jonsson Comprehensive Cancer Center. This drug is now being used to treat women with HER-2 positive breast cancer patients who are, as a result, living longer.

A Word about the Environment and Other Cancer Suspects

Try to avoid the all-or-nothing mentality about research regarding our environment and breast cancer risk. Many have valid links and others still remain controversial. Do your own research and carefully decipher the environmental links to and increased risk of breast cancer. Read the supporting literature and decide for yourself if you need to make changes in your lifestyle and ways of doing things.

 Fact

For more information about environmental exposure, you can refer to a recent study by the Silent Spring Institute and Susan G. Komen for the Cure recently published in *Cancer,* a journal of the American Cancer Society.

One common breast cancer suspect that has been discussed in the media recently is car and truck exhaust, which produces PAHs (polycyclic aromatic hydrocarbons). These toxic products of combustion have been linked to breast cancer in both men and women. The difficulty with some of the environmental exposures is that there is little one can do to avoid them completely. Certainly, the car industry is working on eco-friendlier cars, but this is still in its early stages. Many combustion industries are culprits of air pollution, especially in certain areas of the country, and are associated with higher risk of breast cancer associated with PAHs such as in certain areas in New York State.

Other common environmental sources of toxins are tobacco smoke, food preservatives (especially in fast and prepared foods), some household cleaning products, pesticides, hair dyes, chemicals used by dry cleaners, and many more, seeping into our lives without us knowing the environmental impact and cancer risk. The good news is that we are moving toward an eco-friendly, cleaner environment in which individuals are taking responsibility for a safer world and teaching its principles to the next generation.

APPENDIX A

Glossary

Acupuncture
A Chinese form of medicine, which involves the treatment of disorders by inserting needles into the skin at points where the flow of energy is thought to be blocked, to restore balance and energy.

Adjuvant therapy
Treatment that is added to increase the effectiveness of primary breast cancer treatment. Usually it refers to hormone therapy, chemotherapy, or radiation therapy conducted after surgery to kill any remaining cancer cells and to increase a person's chances of a cure or at least keeping the disease in check.

Angiogenesis
The formation of new blood vessels that aid tumor growth. Certain cancer treatments are geared to blocking new blood vessel growth to help prevent tumor growth.

Antioxidants
A substance that is often used to refer to vitamins, herbs, and foods that help with protecting cells against the effect of free radicals, which have been linked to breast cancer.

Art therapy

A complementary therapy that allows for self-expression in a safe
environment through art and is used to help reduce stress and
increase self-esteem.

Biomarkers

Substances measured either in tumor cells or blood that are used
to guide treatment options. Estrogen and progesterone receptor
status and HER-2 status are considered biomarkers. Identifying
biomarkers will help in the future to promote precision-guided
breast cancer treatment so unnecessary treatment can be
avoided.

BRCA1/BRCA2

Inherited breast cancer genes that are passed on from parent to
child and place women at a higher risk for developing breast or
ovarian cancers compared to women who do not have the gene.

Breast biopsy

A diagnostic procedure in which a piece of tissue and/or cells is
removed to be examined under a microscope by a pathologist.
The tissue or cells are analyzed to look for the presence of cancer
cells, establish tumor grading, and provide more information for
treatment.

Breast cancer margin

The edge of a cancerous sample or lump removed during surgery.
The pathologist examines whether the breast cancer tumor has
clean margins which indicates that most of the cancer cells have
been removed.

Cancer cell

A faulty cell that divides out of control and forms a lump or mass
called a tumor, which can invade and destroy healthy tissue.

Carcinoma

A malignant tumor that starts from epithelial cells in organs. Almost all breast cancers are carcinomas.

CAT scan

Also known as a CT scan. A diagnostic radiological scan in which many x-rays are taken from different angles and then combined by a computer to produce a cross-sectional image of an organ.

Chemo brain

Chemo brain is a recently coined term used to describe the effect chemotherapy has on an individual's ability to process information and to remember. It has been found in men and women who have had high-dose chemotherapy.

Chemotherapy

A systematic approach to cancer treatment that slows down the normal production of blood cells. Cancer cells go through a process of cell division and reproduction. The goal of chemotherapy is to interfere with cancer cells at various stages of their growth.

Core biopsy

Removal of fluid, cells, or tissue with a needle for examination under a microscope, using a thicker needle to remove a cylindrical sample of tissue from a tumor.

Digital mammography

Digital mammography is a method of storing an x-ray image of the breast as a computer image, which helps the radiologists to further interpret the findings as it can be combined with the computer-aided detection (CAD) program.

DNA
A segment of the genes that contain unique information on hereditary characteristics, such as hair color, eye color, or height as well as susceptibility to certain diseases.

Ducts
Ducts are passages in the breast that carry milk to the nipple.

Durable Power of Attorney (DPOA)
A legal document that can only be prepared by an attorney, it appoints a designated person to be a financial representative, usually paying your bills and managing your overall fiscal affairs when you are unable due to illness or other health care issues.

Estrogen receptor status
A hormone-receptor status that indicates whether a tumor is receptive to estrogen, which fuels its growth. The tumor is estrogen-receptor positive if it feeds on estrogen, negative if it doesn't.

Excision biopsy
A method of biopsy in which all or part of a lump is removed by a surgeon for examination.

Fine-needle aspiration
A type of needle biopsy involving the removal of fluid from a cyst or cells from a tumor. A fine (thin) needle is used to reach the cyst or tumor and, with suction, draw up (aspirate) samples for examination under a microscope.

Family Medical Leave Act (FMLA)
A federal law that provides employees with up to twelve weeks of unpaid leave for their own serious illness, the birth or adoption of a child, or care of a seriously ill child, spouse, or parents.

Genetic testing
Testing which involves analysis of your DNA to see if a person has inherited gene changes or mutations that increase your cancer risk.

Healing Touch
Energy work that manipulates energy fields around the body and supports the body's ability to heal with the goal of increasing a sense of well-being.

Health care proxy
A document that designates another person to act on one's behalf in regards to health care decisions if an individual is unable to make his or her own decisions because of illness or other health care issues.

HER-2 positive tumors
A tumor containing a gene that produces a type of receptor that helps cells grow. Cancers that have too much of this receptor gene tend to be more aggressive, but respond to treatment with Herceptin.

Hormone therapy
Treatment with hormones to try to interfere with hormone production or hormone action that promotes cancer growth, or the surgical removal of hormone-producing glands to kill cancer cells or slow their growth. Tamoxiphen is the most common and others include megestrol acetate, aminoglutethimide, androgens, and surgical removal of ovaries.

Immune system
A complex bodily defense system that recognizes and opposes germs (bacteria or viruses) and other foreign material within the body to fight off disease and maintain health and initiates the immune response to fight them.

Incision biopsy
Under local anesthetic, a wedge is surgically removed from the lump for examination.

Inflammatory breast cancer
A type of invasive breast cancer that has spread to the lymphatic vessels in the skin covering the breast. The skin feels warm and may appear thickened. About 1 percent of breast cancers are inflammatory.

In-situ breast cancer
A type of precancerous cell that remains in one location and has not spread to other surrounding tissue.

Invasive breast cancer
Cancer cells that have broken through to surrounding nearby tissue or to distant areas of the body.

Journaling
Writing in a book or journal to express your inner feelings and fears in a safe environment. Journal writing can be a source of healing and strength as you go through cancer treatment.

Lobules
The lobules are the glands that make the milk that then passes through the ducts.

Lump
A tumor in the breast or elsewhere in the body which may be cancerous or not; also referred to as a mass.

Lumpectomy
Surgery to remove a lump from the breast, along with a small amount of surrounding tissue.

Lymph nodes
Bean-shaped nodes under the armpit that carry cleansing lymph fluid through the body's lymphatic system.

Magnetic Resonance Imaging (MRI)
A method of taking pictures of the inside of the body. It differs from x-rays in that it uses a large, powerful magnet to send radio waves through the body, making images appear on a computer screen as well as on film.

Massage
A therapeutic technique of touching and moving the soft tissues of the body.

Mastectomy
Surgery to remove all or part of the breast and sometimes other tissue. An individual may have a full or radical mastectomy (both breasts), or partial mastectomy (one breast).

Meditation
An ancient practice of focusing your mind and thoughts on the present moment. The goal of meditation is to be aware of what is happening in the present moment and meditation requires daily practice to benefit from its stress-reducing effects.

Menopause
A time in a woman's life when monthly cycles of menstruation stop forever and hormone levels decrease. Menopause occurs naturally but it can be brought on abruptly by chemotherapies that destroy ovarian function.

Metastasis
Spread of cancer cells that have migrated to other body sites.

Oncologist
A doctor with special training in the diagnosis, treatment, and care of cancer patients.

Oncotype DX
A gene test that analyzes gene expression patterns that have been linked to more aggressive cancers and a higher risk for recurrence.

Partial mastectomy
Surgery that removes less than the whole breast, taking a part of the breast where the cancer is found and some of the healthy tissue that surrounds the breast.

Radiologist
A doctor with special training in diagnostics and interpreting x-rays and other radiological images and tests.

Reconstructive surgery
Plastic surgery that is done after a mastectomy to rebuild the breast or breasts.

Reiki
A gentle method of hands-on healing that taps into one's energy. *Reiki* is a Japanese word that means "universal life energy."

S-phase
A lab test that shows the percentages of cells that are replicating their DNA. High S-phase division indicates a tumor with cells that are quickly dividing and tend to be more aggressive. A low S-phase is a sign that the tumor is slow growing.

Translational research
Research that moves findings quickly from "the bench to the bedside"—from the research lab to patients. It depends on a collaboration of scientists, researchers, and doctors, and is much more aggressive than traditional research.

Triple-negative tumors
A tumor that has an estrogen-progesterone negative tumor along with a HER-2 negative tumor and so will not benefit from hormone treatments or trastuzumab therapy.

Tumor grade
The histologic grade of the tumor indicates how likely the cancer is to metastasize. (Grade is not to be confused with stage.) The pathologist determines the grade based on visual inspection of the cancer under the microscope.

Ultrasound
A sonogram (a method of imaging the breast with sound waves). It is used as a complement to mammography and is commonly used to target areas for biopsy.

Visualization (guided imagery)
A technique to create a positive mental image used during cancer treatment to promote a sense of well-being.

Yoga
A set of breathing exercises and postures based on a Hindu spiritual discipline that promotes well-being.

APPENDIX B

Resources

Angelou, Maya. *Wouldn't Take Nothing for My Journey Now.* (New York: Random House, 1993).

Begley, Sharon. "Health: Why the War on Cancer Has Fallen Short," *Newsweek*, 15 September 2008, p. 42.

Bender, Sue. *Stretching Lessons.* (San Francisco: Harper San Francisco, 2001).

Buscaglia, Leo. *Love.* (New York: A Fawcett Columbine Book, Published by Ballantine Books, 1972).

Cousins, Norman. *Anatomy of an Illness.* (New York: Norton, 1979; reprint, 2005).

Cukier, Daniel, MD, FACR, Frank Gingerelli, MD, Grace Makari-Judson, MD, and Virginia E. McCullough. *Coping with Chemotherapy and Radiation.* (New York: McGraw-Hill, 2004).

DeAngelis, Michelle. *Get a Life That Doesn't Suck.* (New York: Rodale, 2008).

Dillman, Erica. *The Little Yoga Book.* (New York: Warner Books, 1999).

Dyer, Diana, MS, RD. *A Dietitian's Cancer Story.* (Ann Arbor, Michigan: Swan Press, 2005).

Frankl, Victor. *Man's Search for Meaning.* (Boston, Massachusetts: Beacon Press, 2006).

Griffin, Katherine. "Healing Refuge," *Yoga Journal*, October 2008, p. 90.

Healy, Bernadine, MD. "Unlocking the Secrets of Cancer," *U.S. News & World Report*, 3–10 November 2008, p. 46.

Huang, Lena. "East Meets West: Integrating Traditional Chinese Medicine May Ease Side Effects," *Cure,* Fall Issue, Vol. 7 No. 3 2008, p. 22.

Huddleston, Peggy. *Prepare for Surgery, Heal Faster: A Guide of Mind-Body Techniques.* (Cambridge, Massachusetts: Angel River Press, 1996).

Human, Katy. "Finding Your Compass: New Research and Tools Illuminate the Multiple Treatment Paths Faced by Patients with Early-Stage Invasive Breast Cancer," *Cure,* Fall Issue, Vol. 7 No. 3 2008, p. 45.

Keel, Philipp. *All about Me.* (New York, Broadway Books, 1998).

Kramp, Erin Tierney, Douglas H. Kramp, and Emily P. McKhann. *Living with the End in Mind.* (New York: Three Rivers Press, 1998).

Kübler-Ross, Elisabeth. *On Death and Dying.* (New York: Macmillan, 1969).

Love, Susan M., MD. *Dr. Susan Love's Breast Book.* (Reading, Massachusetts: A Merloyd Lawrence Book, Addison-Wesley Publishing Company, Inc., 1991).

Morgan, Miranda. *My First Book of Pilates.* (New York: Barnes & Noble Books, 2003).

Morrison, Judith H. *The Book of Ayurveda: A Holistic Approach to Health and Longevity.* (New York: A Fireside Book, Simon & Schuster, 1995).

Progoff, Ira, PhD. *At a Journal Workshop: Writing to Access the Power of the Unconscious and Evoke Creative Ability.* (New York: G.P. Putnum's Sons, 1992).

Seligman, Martin E. P., PhD. *Authentic Happiness.* (New York: Free Press, 2002).

Seligman, Martin E. P., PhD. *Learned Optimism.* (New York: Pocket Books, 1998).

Servan-Schreiber, David, MD, PhD. *Anticancer: A New Way of Life.* (New York, Viking, 2008).

Simonton, O. Carl, Stephanie Matthews-Simonton, and James L. Creighton. *Getting Well Again.* (New York: Bantam, 1992).

BREAST CANCER WEBSITE RESOURCES

AMERICAN CANCER SOCIETY
This site provides general cancer information and programs for patients and families, including the publication "What's New in Breast Cancer Research and Treatment?"

www.cancer.org

BREAST CANCER.ORG
This site is run by a nonprofit organization dedicated to providing information and community to those who have been touched by breast cancer.

www.breastcancer.org

CANCER NET.COM
This site is sponsored by the American Society of Clinical Oncology and has a wealth of information for patients.

www.cancer.net/portal/site/patient

TRIAL CHECK.COM
This site is put together by the Coalition of Cancer Cooperative Groups and has excellent information about possible clinical trials.

www.cancertrialshelp.org/trialcheck/default.aspx

APPENDIX C

Breast Cancer and Cancer Organizations

BREAST CANCER ORGANIZATIONS

African American Breast Cancer Alliance, Inc. (AABCA)
www.geocities.com/aabcainc

Avon Breast Cancer Crusade
www.avoncrusade.com

Breast Cancer.org
www.breastcancer.org

The Breast Cancer Fund
www.breastcancerfund.org

Breast Cancer Network of Strength (Formerly Y-ME)
www.networkofstrength.org

Breast Cancer Research Foundation
www.bcrfcure.org

The Department of Defense, Breast Cancer Research Program and Era of Hope
http://cdmrp.army.mil/bcrp

Fight Pink
www.fightpink.org

Kicks Against Breast Cancer
www.kicksagainstbreastcanc.com

Living Beyond Breast Cancer
www.lbbc.org

National Breast Cancer Awareness Month
www.nbcam.org

National Breast Cancer Coalition
www.natlbcc.org

National Breast Cancer Foundation
www.nationalbreastcancer.org

Pink-Link
www.pink-link.org

Recycle for Breast Cancer
www.recycleforbreastcancer.org

The Sister Study
www.sisterstudy.org

Susan G. Komen Breast Cancer Foundation
www.komen.org

Susan Love, MD, Breast Cancer Research Foundation
www.susanlovemd.org

CANCER ORGANIZATIONS

American Cancer Society
www.cancer.org

Gilda's Club Worldwide
www.gildasclub.org

Lance Armstrong Foundation
www.livestrong.org

National Coalition for Cancer Survivorship
www.canceradvocacy.org

National Cancer Institute's Cancer Information Service
www.cancer.gov

Stand Up to Cancer
www.standup2cancer.org

REGIONAL BREAST CANCER ORGANIZATIONS

Alabama: The Breast Cancer Research Foundation of Alabama
(*www.bcrfa.org*)
The Joy to Life Foundation (*www.joytolife.org*)

Alaska: Breast Cancer Focus (*www.breastcancerfocus.org*)

Arizona: Breast Cancer Foundation of Arizona (*www.bcfaz.com*)
The Arizona Institute for Breast Health (*www.aibh.org*)

Arkansas: BreastCare, Arkansas Department of Health
(*www.arbreastcare.com*)

California: California Breast Cancer Organizations
(*www.cabco-org.us*)
California Breast Cancer Research Program (*www.cbcrp.org*)

Colorado: Colorado Breast Cancer Resources Directory
(*www.breastcancercolorado.org*)

Connecticut: Connecticut Breast Cancer Coalition/Foundation
(*www.cbccf.org*)

Delaware: Delaware Breast Cancer Coalition
(*www.debreastcancer.org*)

District of Columbia: Capital Breast Care Center
(*www.capitalbreastcare.org*)

Florida: Florida Breast Cancer Coalition Research Foundation
(*www.fbccrf.org*)

Georgia: Georgia Breast Cancer Coalition (*www.gabcc.org*)

Hawaii: Komen Hawaii (*www.komenhawaii.org*)

Idaho: Angel Care Foundation (*www.angelcarefoundation.org*)

Illinois: The Illinois Breast and Cervical Cancer Program
(*www.cancerscreening.illinois.gov*)

Indiana: Indiana Breast Cancer Awareness Trust
(*www.breastcancerplate.org*)

Indiana Breast and Cervical Cancer Program (*www.uhs-in.org/breast_cervical_cancer.html*)

Iowa: Iowa Breast Cancer Edu-Action (*www.iowabreastcancer.org*)

Kansas: Komen Kansas City (*www.komenkansascity.org*)

Kentucky: Kentucky Breast Cancer Coalition (*www.kybcc.org*)

Louisiana: Hope Chests (*www.hopechests.org*)
Komen New Orleans (*www.komenneworleans.com*)

Maine: Maine Breast Cancer Coalition
(*www.mainebreastcancer.org*)

Maryland: The Red Devils Supporting Breast Cancer Families
(*www.the-red-devils.org*)

Massachusetts: Massachusetts Breast Cancer Coalition
(*www.mbcc.org*)

Michigan: Michigan Breast Cancer Coalition (*www.mibcc.org*)

Minnesota: Breast Cancer Awareness Association of Minnesota
(*www.bcaamn.org*)

Mississippi: Fannie Lou Hamer Cancer Foundation
(*www.fannielouhamercancer.org*)

Missouri: Breast Health Care Center
(*www.breasthealthcarecenter.org*)

Montana: Komen Montana (*www.komenmontana.org*)

Nebraska: Komen Nebraska (*www.komennebraska.org*)

Nevada: Komen Northern Nevada (*www.komennorthnv.org*)
Komen Southern Nevada (*www.komensouthernnevada.org*)

New Hampshire: New Hampshire Breast Cancer Coalition
(*www.nhbcc.org*)

New Jersey: Breast Cancer Resource Center (*www.bcrcnj.org*)
South Jersey Breast Cancer Coalition (*www.southjerseybcc.org*)

New Mexico: New Mexico Breast Cancer Resources
(*www.nmbcr.org*)

**New York: New York State Breast Cancer Support and Education
Network** (*www.nysbcsen.org*)

North Carolina: Breast Cancer Resource Directory of North Carolina
(*www.bcresourcedirectory.org*)
The Carolina Breast Cancer Study (*www.cbcs.med.unc.edu*)

North Dakota: Women's Way (*www.ndhealth.gov/womensway*)

Ohio: Northern Ohio Breast Cancer Coalition Fund (*www.nobcc.org*)
The Breast Cancer Fund of Ohio (*www.bcfohio.org*)

Oklahoma: Oklahoma Breast Care Center (*www.okbreastcare.com*)
Komen Central Oklahoma (*www.komencentralok.org*)

Oregon: Making Memories Foundation
(*www.makingmemories.org*)

Pennsylvania: Pennsylvania Breast Cancer Coalition
(*www.pabreastcancer.org*)

Rhode Island: Gloria Gemma Breast Cancer Resource Foundation
(*www.gloriagemma.org*)

South Carolina: Komen Upstate South Carolina
(*www.komenupstatesc.org*)
Komen Lowcountry (*www.komenlowcountry.org*)

South Dakota: Komen South Dakota
(*www.komensouthdakota.org*)

Tennessee: Tennessee Breast Cancer Coalition (*www.tbcc.org*)

Texas: The Breast Cancer Resource Center (*www.bcrc.org*)

Utah: Komen Salt Lake City (*www.komenslc.org*)

Vermont: Vermont Breast Cancer Conference
(*www.vtbreastcancerconference.org*)
Dragonheart Vermont (*www.dragonheartvermont.org*)

Virginia: Virginia Breast Cancer Foundation (*www.vbcf.org*)
The Virginia Center for Breast Cancer Awareness
(*www.evms.edu/breast-center*)

Washington: Komen Seattle (*www.komenseattle.org*)
Komen Spokane (*www.komenspokane.org*)

West Virginia: Komen West Virginia (*www.komenwv.org*)

Wisconsin: Wisconsin Breast Cancer Coalition
(*www.standupandspeakout.org*)
Breast Cancer Recovery (*www.bcrecovery.org*)

Wyoming: Komen Wyoming (*www.komenwyoming.org*)

APPENDIX D

What to Bring to Your Chemotherapy Appointments

❏ Tote bag, backpack, briefcase—one with several compartments may be helpful to organize your things

❏ Journal

❏ Book you are reading or one that you have wanted to read but have not had the time

❏ Magazines

❏ MP3 player and/or iPod or handheld game

❏ Portable CD player and/or DVD player

❏ Crocheting, knitting, or hobby that you are working on

❏ A friend to keep you company

❏ Healthy snacks to munch on:

- Nuts, almonds, pistachios, pecans, pumpkin seeds, etc.
- Dark chocolate
- Bananas
- Grapes
- Oranges
- Pears

- Power bars or energy bars (You may want to pick ones that support breast cancer such as Luna Bar's Berry Almond.)
- Aluminum water bottle that is eco-friendly so you can have water with you
- Small juice boxes for easy travel
- Gatorade or power water to replenish your electrolytes and fluid
- Trail mix
- Green tea and white tea
- Ginger tea for symptoms of nausea
- Herbal teas
- Jell-O snack cups or pudding cups
- Yogurt for those bouts of diarrhea or to prevent stomach upset
- Oatmeal, cream of wheat
- Fresh fish
- Chicken
- Lean meat (organic preferred)
- Broccoli
- Green leafy vegetables
- Potatoes, sweet potatoes

❑ Bag lunch or breakfast

❑ Lip balm for dry lips

❑ Gum, breath mints, or hard candy for "chemo breath"

❑ Ginger inhaler for nausea (You can often find this at a vitamin and herb store.)

❑ Insurance or hospital registration cards

❑ Names, addresses, and phone numbers of your referral physicians and your primary care doctor

❑ List of your medications and the pharmacy you use

❑ Chemotherapy calendar or daily planner (see printable chemo calendar at *http://guide2chemo.com*)

❑ Shawl or sweater

❑ Pillow or favorite blanket

❑ Water or carbonated drink to help with symptoms of nausea

❑ Laptop to catch up on e-mail or update your facebook or web page

❑ Stationery to send notes or thank-you cards to friends and family

❑ Tape recorder or notebook to write any instructions that are given

Index